Why Ration Health Care?

Why Ration Health Care?

An international study of the United Kingdom, France,
Germany and public sector health care in the USA

Heinz Redwood

CIVITAS: Institute for the Study of Civil Society
London

First published November 2000

CIVITAS: Institute for the Study of Civil Society
The Mezzanine, Elizabeth House
39 York Road
London SE1 7NQ

ISBN 1-903 386-08 X

Typeset by CIVITAS
in New Century Schoolbook

Printed in Great Britain by
The Cromwell Press
Trowbridge, Wiltshire

Contents

The Author

Heinz Redwood works as an author and independent industry consultant.

Trained as a scientist in England, he acquired commercial and marketing experience during four years in Thailand, importing and selling pharmaceutical and chemical products, and subsequently worked for many years in the British pharmaceutical and chemical industry in commercial development and strategic planning.

Since 1982, Dr Redwood has worked as an independent international consultant, specialising in pharmaceutical and healthcare strategy at corporate and industry association level, public policy issues, and the interface between the two.

Dr Redwood was an expert witness in Ottawa at the Senate of Canada hearings on the repeal of compulsory licensing ('C-91') in 1993; and at the House of Commons Health Committee hearings on the National Health Service Drug Budget in London in 1994. He has spoken at pharmaceutical seminars and conferences in Austria, Belgium, Brazil, Canada, Denmark, France, Germany, India, Ireland, Japan, Spain, Sweden, Switzerland, the United Kingdom and the USA.

Heinz Redwood's published studies of pharmaceutical and healthcare topics include: *The Pharmaceutical Industry: Trends, Problems and Achievements*, 1988; *The Price of Health*, Adam Smith Institute, 1989; *Price Regulation and Pharmaceutical Research*, 1993; *New Horizons in India: The Consequences of Pharmaceutical Patent Protection*, 1994; *Brazil: The Future Impact of Pharmaceutical Patents*, 1995; *Pharmapolitics 2000: Key Issues for the Industry*, 1997; 'The Pharmaceutical Price Regulation Scheme: International Perspectives and Millennial Change', in *Should Pharmaceutical Prices be Regulated?*, IEA Health and Welfare Unit, 1997; 'Pharmaceutical cost containment and quality care', *Pharmacoeconomics*, 14, Suppl.1, 1998, 9-14; 'Pharmaceutical reference prices: how do they work in practice?' (with Professor Michael Dickson, University of South Carolina), *Pharmacoeconomics*, 14(5), November 1998, 471-479.

Foreword

Not long ago our politicians used to insist that we must refrain from any talk of 'rationing' and speak instead of 'priority setting'. This pretence that the denial of care is unavoidable is not so common now that the Blair Government has admitted that the NHS falls a long way short of international standards. But just how much health care rationing is there in the UK compared with overseas?

Why Ration Health Care? investigates the withholding and delaying of health care in Germany, France and the publicly-financed schemes in the USA, Medicare and Medicaid. The author finds that the UK stands out from the crowd by a wide margin. Heinz Redwood's study reinforces the suspicion of many informed NHS observers that, even after the substantial influx of funds promised over the next three years, there is no serious prospect of the UK matching the standard of care which is simply taken for granted in nearby France and Germany.

Thanks are due to two anonymous referees for suggesting improvements in the text and to Pfizer for a grant, without which it would not have been possible to carry out fieldwork in Germany, France and America.

David G. Green

Summary

Cost containment in healthcare provision is an aspiration that is common to all systems, whether public or private, motivated by market forces or regulated by central financial controls. Rationing, on the other hand, is far from universal and is often the subject of heated political and academic controversy.

This study attempts to draw a line between cost containment and rationing health care whilst recognising that in many countries there is also a transitional 'grey area' where cost containment is drifting towards rationing (Part I, Chapter 2).

Definitions

Cost containment is defined as the effort to limit a payer's or insurer's healthcare expenditure to a predetermined, usually budgeted or capped sum for a given period of years. It is, above all, a technique of financial control. The impact of cost containment on health care can range from favourable (eliminating waste) through neutral to adverse (costs saved at the expense of the quality of care).

Rationing is less concerned with financial control and more with the allocation and prioritisation of healthcare resources. It is more doctrinaire and interventionist in medical affairs than cost containment.

One or all of four main *symptoms* indicate that rationing is at work (Details: Part I-3):

1. Scarcity of physical resources and a perceived need for their allocation

2. Waiting lists and long waiting times

3. Denial of quality treatment

4. Discrimination between patients regardless of need

Many healthcare experts regard rationing as *inevitable*, without drawing a line between it and cost containment. In rich, industrialised countries, healthcare rationing should be regarded as the exception not the rule. The case of organ transplants is a rare example of *inevitable* rationing, because organ scarcity—not cost—is the principal cause. There is general consensus that rationing of organs is preferable to supply dictated by market forces, even in the USA. However, the problems encountered in rationing organs should serve as a warning to those who regard healthcare rationing as a preferred choice rather than as a last resort (Part I-4).

In the industrialised world, scarcity of *financial* resources for health care is more apparent than real, because it arises not from lack of means but from excessively tight budgeting in relation to demand and unwillingness to pay. These are by-products of the interplay between healthcare politicians and financial controllers. Numerous examples demonstrate that political decisions will overrule budgetary disciplines in health care when the political imperative is sufficiently powerful to stimulate 'willingness to pay'.

International comparisons (Part II-1) reveal a sharp distinction between the United Kingdom and other industrialised countries in health expenditure and resources. When expenditure is measured as a percentage of Gross Domestic Product or *per capita*, and resources by the number of doctors and nurses per head of population, the UK is near the bottom of the ranking lists of OECD member states, in company with Mexico, South Korea and Turkey.

By contrast, Germany and France—whose national income per head of population is similar to that of the UK—rank near the top with the USA. That is true both of public and of private health expenditure. The private contribution to health spending in the UK is *abnormally* low and deprives the system of a degree of flexibility that is helping to relieve the public sector of part of its financial burden in comparable countries.

The most important change in healthcare spending patterns in the industrialised world during the past 20 years has been the gradual convergence of the public/private ratio in the USA from a predominantly private system towards 50/50 balance. In the latter half of the 1990s, this was also accompanied by a stabilisation of health expenditure as a proportion of GDP, as a result of high rates of economic growth and more intensive cost containment of health care.

Although healthcare productivity in the UK is generally high in terms of output and utilisation of its inadequate resources, results in terms of health outcomes often appear inferior, especially for the 65+ age group, when compared with results in France and the USA, and to a lesser extent Germany. Conclusions on outcomes must, however, be regarded as tentative, because they rely on the interpretation of mortality statistics for a range of diseases (Part II-2). Internationally comparable morbidity data (not available) would be more indicative of the health status of living populations.

There is evidence from opinion surveys (Part II-3) that the British public is increasingly dissatisfied with the performance of its healthcare system, more so than the public in France and Germany. This may, however, be attributable in part to the British propensity to let off steam by doing a little grumbling (*The Grumble Hypothesis*). Other evidence shows a high level of satisfaction on the part of British respondents when asked how they feel about the medical treatment that they have *personally* experienced under the National Health Service (NHS).

Personal satisfaction is probably the most persuasive explanation of the continued fervent support by the British electorate of the principle of the NHS as a healthcare monopoly that is largely free at the point of use. Rationing is now observed and admitted to exist, and the British public dislikes it but does not associate it with the conceptual foundations of the NHS (Part II-3).

Part II, Chapters 4-7, examines the rationing situation in the UK, France, Germany and the USA in greater detail. They conclude that, whereas health care in all four countries faces severe financial problems and all are intensifying their efforts to contain costs, the drift towards *rationing* (as defined above) is strongest by far in the UK.

Six 'pathways to rationing' have been identified in the **United Kingdom**:

• almost total dependence of the NHS on funding by taxation

• a chronic state of underfunding

• abnormally low user charges by international standards

• public and political distaste for supplementary forms of health insurance

• the 'efficiency delusion' (that greater efficiency could *solve* the problems of the NHS)

• the British public's modest healthcare expectations by European standards

The resulting rationing climate in the UK is embodied in a National Health Service that is excessively crisis-prone, has unusually long waiting lists and waiting times, and suffers from 'innovation phobia'. None of these symptoms are significant in **Germany**, where rationing is nevertheless the subject of active debate, because most cost-containment measures are either short-lived in their effect or fail. Rationing is not, however, widely perceived as a suitable solution to the problems of a healthcare system that enjoys a very high level of popular support. In practice, there is strong political resistance to actual rationing proposals in Germany when it comes to the crunch.

In **France**, the *dirigiste* tradition of government and officialdom is tackling the persistent financial crisis of public sector health care with a multiplicity of controls, most of which are only briefly effective. There are, however, no clear signs of rationing health care. None of the four symptoms of rationing (see above) is evident in France, although the latest pharmaceutical controls are characteristic of the 'grey area' between cost containment and rationing. The almost universal acceptance of supplementary health insurance on the *'mutualiste'* principle by the French population has given the hard-pressed, high-spending public sector healthcare system in France a degree of financial flexibility which the British system lacks. The French public is satisfied with the results.

In both France and Germany, the financial problems of public sector health care arise mainly from a surplus of resources for populations accustomed to lavish consumption, whereas in the UK the drift towards rationing is caused by a shortage of supply in a system that is basically unresponsive to demand. The impulse to provide more effective health care by *competitive* means is weak and philosophically frowned upon in the three European countries examined.

In the **United States**, the borderline between public sector and private health care is becoming increasingly blurred. In terms of expenditure, the two are now almost in balance. Even more important is their increasing direct collaboration through the medium of managed care which is now responsible for the majority of patients under private employers' insurance as well as under Medicaid in the public sector. Medicare (covering mainly seniors and the severely disabled) is less integrated with managed care but most Medicare patients also have private coverage.

Although Congress failed throughout the twentieth century to resolve the question of universal access to health care in the USA, the 84 per cent of the population that is covered by private or public sector health insurance enjoys generally high standards of care. The competitive principle on which both private insurance and managed care operate, effectively precludes rationing (except under conditions of extreme physical scarcity, as in the case of organ transplants), because the system is basically responsive to demand. The Oregon rationing experiment has not been copied by other states of the union. Instead, vigorous cost containment—the underlying motive for the growth of managed care—tolerates numerous grey-area practices in US health care. When these threaten to get out of hand, the US response is a blend of competition (to attract or hold patients), lawsuits, and a backlash of public opinion that will put strong pressure on Congress to introduce remedial legislation.

Part III focuses on the rationing situation in the United Kingdom. This study is not primarily concerned with reform of the National Health Service but with the persistent rationing *mindset* of that institution and of many opinion leaders in British health care. That mindset is encapsulated in the widely expressed view that 'There Is No Alternative' to rationing.

There *are* alternatives that are workable and capable of producing results at least on a par with those achieved by the NHS and often better, as illustrated by the other countries examined in this study.

Society has changed greatly since the NHS was set up in 1948. The founders' principle of a healthcare monopoly, free at the point of use, needs to be re-examined. Society today is richer, more demanding, more self-indulgent, older with much longer life expectation, and more vulnerable to chronic than to infectious diseases than its counterpart 50 years ago.

Technological advances in medicine (surgery, pharmaceuticals, biotechnology and genomics), have radically transformed the practical scope of health care from the still rather primitive post-Victorian horizon which it had when the NHS was set up. Today, health is the passport to financial and physical independence at working age and in retirement. The extended family, which was still able to look after the old and the sick in 1948, is no longer the norm. 'Empowered' patients (increasingly in single-person households) regard good health as top priority in order to be able to look after themselves.

Healthcare rationing is unsuitable and inconsistent with social realities and trends: nothing else is rationed in rich, industrialised countries under normal circumstances. The alternatives to rationing health care comprise:

• reconsideration of the principle of providing 'free' health care for all at the point of use by reverting to the original purpose of 'solidarity', which was to provide adequate care for those who are unable to provide it for themselves

• modifying the monopoly concept of healthcare provision by diversification of funding and diversification of choice

• encouraging greater individual responsibility for health

Of these, international experience demonstrates that the first two are feasible, capable of producing satisfactory results and (as illustrated by Switzerland) compatible with the European principle of solidarity without having to resort to rationing. Greater individual responsibility for health is a concept that is not yet widely accepted against a historical background of *cradle to grave* provision of health care by the public sector, but greater patient *empowerment* also implies greater individual responsibility.

In the United Kingdom, the rationing mindset has helped to ossify outdated attitudes towards the National Health Service. The National Plan of July 2000 will help to relieve the worst manifestations of rationing in the short term by injecting substantial additional funds into the system. That has been widely welcomed by professional and public opinion. In the medium term, however, the National Plan risks running out of steam, because it fails to react to changes in society.

Complacently, the National Plan rejects the experience of other countries with the extraordinary assertion that their systems 'do not provide a better route to health care'. This misses the point. All systems are imperfect. Neither social insurance, nor tax funding, nor private health insurance, nor supplementary coverage *alone* will provide the solution to the problems of healthcare funding and performance. In effect, there is no such thing as The Solution. One size no longer fits all, if indeed it ever did. The complexity of modern society demands a multiplicity of partial solutions for different circumstances, flexible enough to change as circumstances alter. The adherence of the National Plan to system purity implies a risk that it will in practice be no more than a 'stopgap' measure in the ineluctable march of British health care towards rationing.

What is needed is a less doctrinaire, less politically correct and more flexible approach involving plurality of funding and choice, as well as the adaptation of some of the more successful features of international experience to British conditions and preferences. Today, there is an evident lack of political will by both government and the British public to move in these directions.

To change public and political opinions that are set in concrete is never easy. Yet it needs to be attempted, because rationed health care in the hands of a 'monopoly that is free at the point of use' will not be able to cope with social change and popular demand for health care in the twenty-first century.

Part I

Rationing and Cost Containment

Introduction

We put too much faith in systems and look too little to men.

Disraeli

There is a paradox in healthcare rationing. In theory, it looks to patients as people in the name of equity, fairness and justice. In practice, rationing puts 'too much faith in systems' and tends to forget about patients as individuals. In the theology of rationing, people are paramount as long as they behave collectively. An individual sticks out like a sore thumb.

Real patients become regrettable obstacles to the orderliness of rationing. Increasingly, they are asserting their patients' rights. Those who have dollars (francs, pounds, etc) brandish them. The diplomats among patients wheedle their way to the head of the queue. The organised patients' movement threatens to vote for the other side at the next election ... and vast numbers of patients suffer in silence.

The industrialised world is ageing and the demand for health care is rising. Scientific and technological advances in surgery, immunology, pharmaceuticals and genomics are ushering in an innovative burst that will be more fundamental than the 'wonder drug' era of 1935-1960.

Patients will want the benefits of innovation as well as the best in more traditional forms of health care. In the battle between *insatiable* demand and *limited* resources, healthcare rationing is *inevitable*.

Perhaps we should pause at this point.

Is demand really *insatiable*? How *limited* are the resources of rich countries?

And might the *inevitability* of healthcare rationing actually be *evitable*?

This study attempts to throw light on complex problems by analysing the position and developments in four industrialised countries with different medical cultures, different healthcare systems, but similar perceptions of conflict between healthcare demand and financial resources. The common denominator between the United Kingdom, France, Germany and public sector health care in the USA is an acknowledged need for cost containment and expenditure control. These are, indeed, *inevitable*, indisputable and undisputed. What is unclear is whether cost containment and expenditure control are synonymous with rationing. Alternatively, is there a borderline, or perhaps a grey area, that separates them?

Part I explores the borderline between cost containment and rationing.

Part II compares the current situation and trends internationally.

Part III examines the battleground of rationing between the opposing forces of pugnacious *TINA* (*There Is No Alternative*) and thoughtful *DORA* (*Discover Other Realistic Answers*), with particular emphasis on the United Kingdom where Tina is currently beating the life out of Dora.

1

The R-word in Healthcare Politics

Rationing is a technique of distributing scarce resources. Bureaucrats like the orderliness of rationing because it eases the problem of administering healthcare budgets. Academics enjoy the celebrity of fathering new theories of healthcare rationing with or without technicalities attached. Many governments would like to ration health care for financial reasons, but hesitate to do so overtly for fear of electoral repercussions. The majority of physicians, carers and other providers as well as patients are guarded in their view of rationing.

In the UK, awareness of rationing increased markedly during the 1990s. An analysis of three public opinion surveys between 1991 and 1994 suggested that 'the public believes that rationing in the NHS *is a reality* (Gallup 1994) but that it *need not be* (Gallup 1991, MORI 1993)'.[1] In other words, people question the *inevitability* of healthcare rationing.

Rationing Is A Political Process[2]

The noble sentiments of rationing theory—its objectives being equity and fairness—are largely lost in the turmoil of healthcare politics. There, the resonance of the R-word is mainly pejorative. Many voters feel that rationing somehow deprives them of their rights. Having paid taxes or social insurance contributions, they feel entitled to demand what they have paid for, especially if they are not getting it.

Consequently, the R-word carries potent emotive undertones that can make voters—politically speaking—sick. In Europe, healthcare 'rationing' can tune the political atmosphere in roughly the same manner as 'socialised medicine' does in the USA. The words 'socialised medicine' reek of government interference and the curtailment of medical freedom. In Europe, 'socialised medicine' would be called 'solidarity in health care'—a cherished principle whereby society will help those who are incapable of helping themselves. 'Rationing', on the other hand, has until recently been banned from the vocabulary of European healthcare politics. In effect, its connotations are not very different from those of 'socialised medicine' in the USA: government interference, bureaucratic allocations, and curtailment of medical freedom which puts you, the patient, at the mercy of faceless, impersonal rationers.

Yet in the UK, during the second half of the 1990s, the 'R-word' began to be aired cautiously in political circles, like a dangerous dog being taken for a walk on a short lead. Experts with impeccable credentials began openly to advocate rationing. The aggressive pit bull terrier was being transformed into an elegant poodle and groomed for exhibition. Meanwhile, in France and Germany, rationing in the UK was being discussed in hushed tones as a cautionary tale of the dreadful state of affairs one could get oneself into if one handled public sector health care *à l'anglaise*.

Priority Setting

To ease the pain, rationing began to be called 'priority setting'—a misnomer and a euphemism with appeal to healthcare politicians who could now avoid having to call a spade a spade. 'I am glad to say that I have never seen a spade', declared the excessively healthy Gwendolyn Fairfax in Oscar Wilde's *The Importance of Being Earnest*. Advocates of rationing disguised as priority setting, please note. There is a world of difference between being an expert in priority setting and a patient who has to endure *non*-priority status under rationing.

In reality, 'priority setting' is of course inevitable. The process of efficient and effective management necessarily involves the setting of priorities in order to avoid dissipation of effort or losing sight of goals. That is true of government, services, industry, opera houses and football clubs, in short of any form of organised activity, including health care:

> Priorities have to be set in all healthcare systems whatever their level of expenditure and regardless of the methods of financing and delivery that are adopted. The nature of the choices that have to be made and the locus of these choices does vary between systems but the inevitability of priority setting is universal.[3]

Priority setting is not *per se* synonymous with rationing, but it forms part of the rationing process, just as putting your foot on the brake forms part of the process of driving a motor vehicle. Priorities can be set without rationing, but rationing cannot be carried out without setting priorities.

Cost Containment

The same could be said of cost containment: it is a necessary component of rationing, but costs can be contained without resorting to rationing (see Part I-2 'Crossing the Border'). Politically, cost containment is an expression that is less inflammatory than rationing. Voters may be emotional, but they are not short of common sense. There is a fairly wide consensus that containing healthcare costs 'within reason' is a necessity and a sign that expenditure is being managed efficiently.

Thus cost containment can have positive connotations in the voter's mind, especially if someone else is made to pay, for example (in Health-Politics-Speak) the Excessively Profitable Pharmaceutical Industry. Here, the link between today's profit and tomorrow's innovation to the benefit of health care is either imperfectly understood or deliberately ignored.

Cost containment works in short time-cycles. It looks for immediate results and tends to overclaim these for political advantage. Unlike rationing, the claims of cost containment are often taken at face value and in isolation of longer-term repercussions. As soon as one measure has run its course, another can be introduced. In healthcare politics, cost containment is a renewable resource.

This raises two interesting questions: firstly, does rationing try to hide in the protective embrace of cost containment? The answer is yes. The phenomenon is known in Germany as 'invisible rationing'. Secondly, where is the borderline between the two? At what point do politically acceptable methods of cost containment become practices to which the dreaded 'R-word' has to be attached? The following chapter will explore the borderline issue.

2

Crossing the Border

What Is Cost Containment?

Briefly, cost containment is the effort to limit a payer's or insurer's healthcare expenditure to a predetermined, usually budgeted or capped sum, for a certain number of years.

In the public sector, (funded directly or indirectly by national, federal, or state authorities, or otherwise publicly accountable), budgetary or cash limits are set centrally. In the private sector, insurers, managed care and other relevant bodies, plan their expenditure competitively. All payers try to contain costs. Most of them will seek to supply adequate or superior healthcare services within budgetary limits.

In practice, often 'something has to give': quality, the budget, or both. Whether payers can succeed in providing or securing quality care within pre-set limits will depend on many factors:

A. Has the budget been set at a realistic level in terms of quantity, quality and cost?

B. Are the required medical resources (institutional, ambulatory, pharmaceutical etc) available and affordable?

C. Is the medical performance of the organisation adequate, efficient and effective?

D. Is expenditure under effective management control?

E. Is clinical performance monitored with reliable data collection and feedback?

F. (in private health care) Are insurers and providers capable of attracting and holding patients with budgeted levels of expenditure?

The answers to these questions will indicate either that there is a need for more effective cost containment (questions D and E) or will point the way to more fundamental probing: 'If not, why not?' (questions A, B, C and F), for example:

Why is the budget unrealistic?

Why is there an imbalance between supply and demand?

Why is performance sub-standard?

Why are we losing ground to competitors?

This form of enquiry will either lead straight back to questions C and D (poor management, lack of feedback) or indicate deficiencies in A and B: excessively tight budgeting and/or inadequate resources.

Negative answers to A and B are fundamental pre-conditions for *rationing*—a last resort when the system has failed (sometimes for good reasons) to achieve financial targets and lacks the resources to bring supply into equilibrium with demand.

Imbalances Between Supply And Demand

There is often a conflict between A and B. Centrally-controlled public sector health care is concerned above all with question A: effective budgetary control. It is relatively insensitive to demand (point B) unless healthcare politicians twist their officials' arms in response to the pressure of public opinion, organised patients' advocacy groups, or the proximity of elections. These are political emergencies that call for temporary relaxation of budgetary control and firm denial of rationing.

Private health care, on the other hand, can have a dual structure: 'for profit' and 'not for profit'. Both operate competitively and, if they wish to be successful, must be responsive to the demand side of the health-care market.

There is an acute need for cost containment in both public and private health care. However, when the public sector is driven into a corner it will if necessary overrule demand by rationing supply. In the private sector, by contrast, failure to respect demand is competitively suicidal and rationing—unless practised mildly and 'invisibly' in grey areas—is no solution.

Public and private sector health care are, in some ways, complementary in their motivation and reaction to imbalances between supply and demand. The public sector resorts to controls and, ultimately, rationing. The private sector adjusts prices, the healthcare palette, and the reimbursement menu.

The Rationale Of Rationing

What is the purpose of rationing? For a start, let us dismiss the idea that rationing health care resembles food rationing and clothes rationing in World War II or petrol rationing during the oil crises of the 1970s. It does not. These measures were concerned with distributing equal maximum quantities of the scarce 'necessities of life' to everyone. There was never any question of rationing caviar and champagne. If you wanted those, you paid—assuming you could afford to do so.

The distribution of equal maximum quantities (picturesquely, two ounces of butter and one egg per person per week) would be nonsensical in health care: two surgical operations per patient per decade? Fortunately, not everyone will need a heart bypass, a kidney graft, or beta-interferon, to name just three treatments that are frequently mentioned in a rationing context.

The crux of rationing is that not everyone who needs treatment will get it. When healthcare supply falls short of demand, agonising choices have to be made—agonising, at least, for doctors and patients. Such rationing may be unavoidable, as for example, with organ grafts where there are long-standing donor shortages.

Physical shortages are, however, merely the tangible tip of an ideological iceberg. Even if the money is there, the UK has a long-standing ideological hang-up about tapping it from all available sources, private as well as public. When it comes to the crunch, rationing is the preferred solution. Indeed, its more fervent advocates have repeatedly proclaimed rationing as *inevitable*; in other words, the *only* solution.

Definitions Of 'Rationing'

Various definitions, taken from recent literature, will illustrate how far *healthcare* rationing has strayed from the traditional concept of equity. The fact that many of the quotations are British is attributable to the UK's persistent preoccupation with the subject.

i)   'Allocating resources when their supply is limited' (Geursen)[1]

ii)   'Managing scarcity' (Spiers)[2]

iii) 'A process ...that decides who should get what' (New and Le Grand)[3]

iv)   'The displacement of the interests of one group of patients by another' (Spiers)[4]

v)   'How many of a given intervention will be provided, to whom, at what cost, and under what circumstances' (Cooper)[5]

vi)   *Denial, Delay and Dilution* (Green & Casper)[6]

vii) 'Giving patients less demonstrably effective health care than might be desirable in the absence of resources constraints (and from which they would benefit)' (Klein)[7]

viii) *'Die künstliche Verknappung eines durchaus vorhandenen Angebots'*
      'The artificial curtailment of supply when it is actually available' (Cueni)[8]

ix) 'Rationing is not uniform in its effects—it has most impact on those kinds of care which need the most new resources' (Bosanquet)[9]

These quotations make up a kaleidoscope of related themes, progressing from the causes of rationing to its consequences.

Limited resources and the need to manage scarcity are basic preconditions. There is no need to resort to rationing when supplies are ample, although even that can happen when financial resources are perceived, rightly or wrongly, to be scarce (see quotation viii).

The next phase is represented by quotations iii, iv and v: 'Who Gets What?' This is where healthcare rationing tends to go off the rails, because the collective decision on paper runs counter to real life medical decision making in hospitals and physicians' offices. Patients are individuals and egotists. I may accept the need for rationing in principle—but, doctor, please, look at the state I'm in! 'Who Gets What' in health care is a planner's dream that can quickly become a physician's cross and a politician's nemesis, especially if the rationing plan does not spring from physical shortages but from financially inadequate budgets.

The last four quotations epitomise what might be called the 'let down' element in healthcare rationing. Care is being denied, delayed and diluted (vi). Patients no longer receive the best treatment (vii) in spite of government assurances that everyone will get all the medical care they need. Supply can become irrelevant when demand is being forcibly cut back by rationing (viii), not for medical but for financial reasons. Finally, patients who need innovative treatments are hit hardest (ix) because innovation is expensive and often a prime target for rationing.

Slipping Across The Border

In the literature on the subject, there is prolific overlap between what might be called genuine rationing (as illustrated by the nine quotations, above) and the wider area of cost containment and expenditure restraint. How can one distinguish between rationing and cost containment?

It is difficult to be precise, except at the extreme ends of the spectrum. In between, there is a grey area where rationing and cost containment possess certain common features which makes it hard to tell them apart. There, healthcare management can glide gradually and almost imperceptibly from cost containment into rationing.

Cost containment, as already described, is in essence a tool of budgetary control with short time-horizons. Its steering mechanisms are largely financial with no precise clinical objectives other than the maintenance of good medical practice consistent with prudent spending.

That is not to say that cost containment measures will lack medical impact. On the contrary, that impact can be substantial and much of it will obey the law of unintended consequences.

Example: Pharmaceutical price regulation tends to diminish price competition. It actually helps to preserve the controlled price long after the relevant patents have expired, and inhibits the growth of cheaper generic versions. Thus, generic prices are low in the free-pricing market of the USA and their market penetration is high. Conversely, in France where drug prices are tightly controlled, they tend to remain stable after patent expiry, and generic competition has until now been feeble. The intention of French price regulation of drugs is cost containment. There is no rationing objective. Indeed, France is renowned for its rapid acceptance and high-volume prescribing and consumption of costly innovative drugs.

Rationing, at the other extreme, will intervene directly in medical decisions by selecting patients for treatments and treatments for patients under conditions of perceived or actual scarcity of resources. Most rationing is financially motivated but, in its purest form, rationing is a response to physical shortages.

Example: The rationing of organ transplants in North America and Europe is conditioned by chronic shortage of organs, not by cost-containment targets. It is perhaps the most convincing example of 'inevitable' rationing. The debate focuses not on *whether* organ grafts should be rationed but *how*. The criteria for patient selection and organ allocation are predominantly medical. Rationing is preferable to the alternative: a black market in organs. (For more detailed analysis and discussion, see case study in Part I-4).

When tightness of *financial* resources is used to justify tough cost containment, one of the tell-tale signs that *rationing* is at work is medical discrimination between patients 'by order from above'. Rationing will override a physician's judgment of what is best for an individual patient. Orchestrated by health economists and implemented by centralised bureaucracy, the process uses *non*-medical administrators to authorise the doctor's proposed treatment.

Here, we find ourselves on the threshold of a grey area. 'Prior authorisation' may be no more than a cost-containment measure designed as a deterrent for doctors who want to avoid the time-wasting tedium of having to fill in forms. Authorisation may be little more than rubber-stamping the forms of those doctors who are determined enough to overcome their inertia. On the other hand, when prior authorisation is applied rigorously, we are close to rationing. We may, indeed, already have slipped across the border.

3

Symptoms and Tools:
A Spectrum of White, Grey and Black

The grey (or transitional) area between cost containment and rationing is elusive: by definition, grey areas are neither black nor white but a mixture of the two in a variety of shades. A useful approach may be to classify observed symptoms in each of the three areas.

'White' Symptoms: Cost Containment That is Not Rationing
i)   Price regulation
ii)   Medical guidelines for 'appropriate' prescribing and for the use of medical technology
iii)   Monitoring of prescription patterns
iv)   Physicians as gatekeepers
v)   Reimbursement regulations based on medical criteria
vi)   Patients' co-payment
vii)   Avoidance of waste
viii) Elimination of surplus resources

Grey Area
i)   Prior authorisation of treatment by—or by order of—*non*-medical personnel
ii)   Exclusion from reimbursement
iii)   Cash limits, volume or benefit caps
iv)   Quality problems and below-standard outcomes
v)   Level of complaints
vi)   Absence of competition
vii)   'Invisible' rationing

'Black' Symptoms: Rationing
i)   Scarcity of physical resources

ii)   Waiting lists and waiting times

iii) Denial of quality treatment

iv)   Discrimination between patients regardless of need

What About Shortage Of Financial Resources?

Shortage of funds obviously plays a major role in all cost-containment activities. Yet it has been excluded from the 'symptoms' of rationing, because it is apt to be advanced as a *pretext*. By and large, rich industrialised countries can afford whatever they prioritise. There does not appear to be a shortage of funds for military operations when we are determined to fight. Are we sufficiently determined to fight for health? What is in question is not our spending power but our *willingness to pay*—and that is not primarily a financial but a *political* decision.

Budgets: healthcare budgets, drug budgets, annual budgets, five-year budgets, or capped budgets are administrative vehicles for expenditure control. They represent what those who determine the size of the budget are willing to spend, not what the country can afford. It is of course true to say that *budget holders* cannot 'afford' to exceed the prescribed limits without incurring their masters' displeasure and possibly losing their jobs. The fact that expenditure is tightly controlled is, however, unrelated to what is or is not affordable. Affordability in rich countries is not limited by budgets. It is a variable quantity, dictated by political events and moulded by political pressures.

How else can we explain the fact that the French authorities, whose mastery of the mechanisms of financial control is legendary, decided some years ago that French doctors would now be allowed to prescribe the latest anti-HIV drugs *'outside* their practice budgets'? This happened after months of fruitless negotiations about pricing and reimbursement during which the authorities had insisted that the public sector could not afford to pay for these innovative drugs.

Again, how can we explain Germany's failure in the summer of 1999 to implement a radical pharmaceutical rationing proposal by the Federal Association of Sickness Fund Physicians (*Kassenärztliche Bundesvereinigung*)? It was intended to help doctors to keep within their 1999 prescribing budgets. However, the Federal Minister of Health intervened to veto it (see Part II-6). Budget or no budget, it was too hot a political potato.

And, on a far grander scale, how is one to explain the British government's sudden decision in March 2000 that it can now afford to raise healthcare expenditure as a percentage of GDP from one of the lowest places in the European ranking list to the EU average? This after years of telling the electorate that 'We don't need to and can't afford it'. What has changed except the political climate—and with it, willingness to pay?

In short, when organising financial resources and cash flow management for public sector health care, the system relies on budgeting or capping. The budget holder who administers expenditure may complain with some justification of 'a shortage of financial resources' and consider certain medical goods and services 'unaffordable'. To take such declarations at face value is to misunderstand the dynamics of affordability in the public sector.

The Tools Of Cost Containment And Rationing

Leaving aside financial resources, every healthcare system in the industrialised world uses a mixture of 'white' (cost containment) and 'grey' tools to achieve its targets. Some tools are also tinged with 'black' (rationing). These control tools will now be examined in turn.

'White' Controls

i) *Price regulation*

This has proven a relatively ineffective tool of cost containment as a substitute for a competitive market (for example, for pharmaceuticals), but has achieved notable results when applied within institutions such as diagnosis-related groups (DRGs) or contractually by negotiation of capitated fees. Holding down prices and fees is evidently an attempt to contain expenditure. Whether regulation can achieve this more successfully in health care than negotiation and market mechanisms is an open question.

ii) *Clinical guidelines*

Guidelines for appropriate prescribing and the use of medical technology are spreading. They are acceptable and may be desirable as long as 'appropriate' is not simply a smokescreen for 'cheapest' and provided the guidelines allow for the needs of the individual and exceptional patient. This is particularly important for conditions where individual responses to standard drug treatment can vary dramatically: mental diseases, migraine, and prescribing for the elderly are well recognised examples.

iii) *Monitoring of doctors' prescribing 'profiles'*

The main objective here is to spot 'outliers' whose prescribing volume, choice and expenditure are abnormally costly after allowing for the demographic and morbidity characteristics of the practice. 'Profiling' is widely adopted, both in the public sector and in managed care. It is a rational management tool for controlling expenditure.

iv) *The use of physicians as gatekeepers*

Gatekeeping confines a patient's direct access to the GP with whom that patient has registered. Only the gatekeeper can refer that patient to a specialist. It also stops 'shopping around', i.e. seeking a second, third, and fourth opinion from other GPs or specialists without referral—a common phenomenon in France and Germany. Gatekeeping is an accepted practice in US managed care and in the British National Health Service. France is beginning to encourage it by voluntary registration of patients with a *médecin référent* (referring doctor). In Germany, it remains experimental.

Gatekeeping is a logical tool of cost containment where resources are strained because it obstructs wilful overconsumption of medical skills.

v) *Reimbursement rules based on medical criteria**

Regulations governing the admittance of healthcare goods and services to reimbursement are universal both in the public and in the private sector. Their purpose is to cover the cost incurred by patients with due regard for cost containment. Reimbursement may be 100 per cent, or payers may list those goods and services which they will reimburse partially, and exclude others altogether (see 'Grey Area', ii, p. 21).

The most common criterion for total reimbursement is 'medical necessity'. This normally includes life-saving drugs, visits to doctors and hospitalisation (other than the so-called 'hotel' expenses). Drugs, in particular, may be listed on formularies or positive lists (i.e. entitled to reimbursement), usually following negotiations about prices or discounts as a condition of listing. That is the case in France and in managed care in the USA. In the UK, a somewhat ambiguous situation has been created by the setting up of the National Institute for Clinical Excellence (NICE) which has no role in pricing but can recommend in favour or against prescribing drugs after investigating their cost-effectiveness. In Germany, the establishment of a positive list has been mooted, suspended, and re-mooted repeatedly throughout the last decade.

The question of 'medical necessity' is determined by clinical appraisal, for example by Pharmacy and Therapeutics (P&T) Committees in US hospitals and managed care, and by the *Commission de la*

---

* The expression 'reimbursement', as used here, denotes either no payment by the patient, or the patient pays but is subsequently reimbursed

Transparence in France, which assesses the SMR (*Service Médical Rendu* or medical value) of drugs.

When 'medical necessity' is not established with certainty, partial or conditional reimbursement may be granted, either as a percentage of costs (in France and a number of other European countries) or up to a predetermined limit such as a given number of tablets per week or per month as in US managed care.

This type of reimbursement control tries to combine cost containment with 'good medical practice'. In its more militant forms, it can be said to enter the grey area between cost containment and rationing.

vi) *Patients' co-payment*

The most common forms of co-payment require patients who are covered by health insurance to pay a deductible before being reimbursed for additional costs, and/or paying additionally at the point of use. This may involve *per diem* charges for hospitalisation, fixed charges for visits to GPs, prescription charges for drugs, or 'excess' thresholds for total medical costs.

The main objective of co-payment is not to reduce consumption —which may or may not be the result—but to shift costs from the insurer to the patient.

Until now, co-payment has been relatively low as a proportion of cost, both in US managed care and in European public sector health care. Most European systems exempt certain groups of patients altogether. These may include those below a certain income level, pensioners, children, pregnant women, and patients with life-threatening or multiple diseases. In the UK, 83 per cent of all prescriptions have for some years been exempt from the prescription charge. This has largely defeated its original purpose.

Co-payment is contentious, both medically and politically. It is unpopular with patients, although a substantial rise in German co-payment for drugs by the Kohl Administration in its last year (and since partially reversed by the Schroeder Administration) caused remarkably little political uproar. Like the dog in the Sherlock Holmes mystery,[1] most patients failed to bark.

Whether co-payment causes patients to cut down on *necessary* medical care is also in dispute. In Europe, moderate increases in co-payment could serve to remind patients that they also have some responsibility for their own health, thereby diminishing the 'moral hazard' inherent in total health insurance coverage.

vii) *Avoidance of waste*

Evidently, to avoid waste is wholly desirable and will help to contain costs. Waste in health care means unnecessary, needlessly costly, obsolete and ineffective treatments. It means over-prescribing as well as failure to secure the patient's compliance with prescribing instructions and failure to complete necessary treatments. At the other extreme, prolonging a state of ill health by under-prescribing or undue delay will cause higher longer-term expenditure arising from the need to treat consequential health damage.

There is always scope for reducing and avoiding waste in health care, but there is also a tendency to over-estimate real potential savings from its elimination. Conversely, consequential problems from under-treatment and delay tend to be under-estimated or ignored, because they are difficult to express in budget language.

In countries where medical culture favours treatments that are regarded as ineffective or obsolete elsewhere, attempts to make a clean sweep of such treatments have run into heavy weather politically. In Germany, for example, there have been prolonged and passionate disputes over the reimbursement of homeopathic medicines and about other, so-called *Umstrittene Medikamente* (medicines of disputed utility). The latter still form a significant part of German drug expenditure by the sickness funds. Resistance, not just to their de-listing from reimbursement but to published criticism of these products has led to court cases and even temporary censorship.

Many doctors believe that the *placebo* effect has its uses in modern medical practice, and that an all-out attack on it would not contain costs but increase them as a result of switches in prescribing to more expensive medicines. This, in turn, may produce better health outcomes and actually save money. Even 'war on waste' can be subject to the law of unintended consequences.

The attack on waste is one solution, not *the* solution, to the problem of rising expenditure. The scope for effective waste reduction varies from country to country. In the USA, dramatic savings have been achieved by managed care but, after 'picking the low-hanging fruit' the drive began to lose momentum, or else it advanced at the expense of quality. This in turn produced a stormy political backlash against managed care in the late-1990s, with strong pressure for legislation to protect patients' rights.

In France and Germany, 'wasteful' health care remains a recognised problem and there is undoubtedly scope for substantial savings, especially in hospital management. The obstacles are political, with energetic resistance by doctors' lobbies and by local interests who shout 'NIMBY!' (Not In My Back Yard) in response to proposals to rationalise the provision of hospital care.

In the UK, despite vigorous denials by bureaucrats in search of cost containment, the scope for waste reduction, whilst never negligible, is modest. The National Health Service is widely recognised as an organisation of above-average efficiency by the standards of public sector health administration. Its problems arise more from under-provision than from squandering resources.

When the British Audit Commission examined the scope for more rational prescribing in the NHS in 1994, it identified 'total longer-term potential' for savings as about 14 per cent of the total prescription drug bill in England and Wales at that time. It added somewhat ominously that 'it will take time and major behavioural change to achieve this level of saving'.[2] Considering that prescription drugs made up only 12.6 per cent of total NHS expenditure in 1994, the 'longer-term potential' from more rational prescribing may be estimated as roughly 1.7 per cent of NHS spending eventually and after 'major behavioural change'. Without belittling the desirability of more rational prescribing, the prospects for cost containment by this route in England and Wales could hardly be described as volcanic.

viii) *Elimination of surplus resources*

The resources in question include physicians, nurses, auxiliary personnel, hospitals, beds, and medical technology.

For savings to be achievable, there must be a surplus of such resources in the first place. This largely leaves the UK as a *non-runner*, because most of these resources are not over-supplied but scarce in the NHS.

A surplus of doctors certainly exists in France and Germany, and action has been taken in both countries to restrict or reduce entry into the profession compared with an excessive inflow in past decades. The results are slow to materialise.[3] Meanwhile, a surplus of doctors is seen as one of the causes of over-treatment as they scramble to maintain or raise patient numbers and earnings. Powerful medical lobbies and the absence of managed care mechanisms to counter overspending have slowed French and German progress in eliminating surplus resources. The same applies, for reasons given above, to institutional establishments and hospital beds.

In the USA, on the other hand, managed care, DRGs and competition have reduced surplus resources substantially without, however, correcting the underlying imbalances. These are: an excess of resources for the insured; reasonably good resources for beneficiaries of public sector health care; and serious shortcomings in the resources devoted to the so-called 'near-poor'. These include patients who are not old enough to enrol in Medicare, not poor enough or sufficiently handicapped to qualify for Medicaid, not covered for health care by employers, and unable to afford private health insurance.

Grey Area Controls

These represent practices that go beyond 'normal' cost containment and may contain elements of rationing, but fall short of full-blown rationing.

i) *Prior authorisation of treatment by non-medical personnel*

To obtain a clinical second opinion is the traditional way for doctor and patient to resolve uncertainty over treatment decisions. 'Prior authorisation' is different: it is not seeking an opinion but asking for permission to treat with reimbursement. It may be required for listed (usually costly) treatments. Its purpose is only partly medical; the other (often predominant) purpose is financial. The system smells of financial priorities when prior authorisation is left in the hands of *non*-medical organisations or of doctors who are obliged to abide by their decisions.

Yet prior authorisation falls short of outright rationing, because the procedure usually has a clinical purpose, too. The medico-financial dilemma of prior authorisation was poignantly illustrated by the notorious 'Child B' case in the UK in the mid-1990s.

Child B suffered from acute myeloid leukaemia. A first bone-marrow transplant was covered by the NHS but was only temporarily effective. The health authority then withheld its consent (i.e. coverage) for a second such intervention. The father of Child B sued the health authority, accusing it of allowing financial motives to prevail over medical considerations. The health authority's defence was that it had exercised reasonable medical judgment in concluding that the chances of success were minimal. It won the case. Next, a private donation enabled Child B to undergo a novel and experimental form of treatment which was successful ... for a while. A year later, Child B died.

Medically, the sequence of events represented a succession of grey areas. Legally, the health authority was vindicated. Ethically, it was on somewhat less certain ground. Had the proposed intervention been cheap or cheaper, would the authority still have refused to pay? At what price might there have been a change of mind? Or was medical judgment absolutely the only consideration? If so, how would that judgment have appeared had Child B survived the subsequent privately donated intervention? That is speculation. The fact is, the authority's judgment was proved right by events. All along, however, decision making was hanging by a grey thread.

ii) *Exclusion from reimbursement*

As long as the concept of 'medical necessity' was relatively unambiguous, exclusions from reimbursement were not particularly controversial. Although interested parties protested vigorously when the exclusion of spa 'cures' was mooted in Germany, the case for de-listing these sojourns (uncharitably dubbed 'paid holidays at a *Kurhaus*') appeared clear-cut, at least outside Germany.

Similarly, the exclusion of over-the-counter drugs (in most countries), of cosmetic surgery, and (more arguably but less argued because the public did not rise in sympathy) sex-change operations has been widely accepted as outside the range of the public sector's obligation to honour the solidarity principle. In the private sector, it is of course market forces that determine the majority of such decisions.

Much more controversial have been the decisions by a number of European countries to exclude dental treatment and optical goods and services. Are these not 'medically necessary'? The consequences of postponing or forgoing a dental check-up or an eye test can be serious. Prevention is strongly advocated by health professionals. On the other hand, many believe that individuals should take greater personal responsibility for preventive measures. Should they not pay for optical and dental care when they can evidently afford holidays abroad, consumer durables, alcohol and tobacco?

The underlying motive for excluding 'eyes and teeth' is cost containment. To the extent that 'medical necessity' is being selectively ignored, however, grey-area precedents are being set.

The greyest area of all is that of the so-called 'lifestyle' drugs. This is both a misnomer and not an entirely new phenomenon. For example, for decades some countries (including Germany and the Netherlands) have refused to reimburse oral contraceptives—which are prescription drugs—on the grounds that pregnancy is not a disease and that, therefore, the pill is not 'medically necessary'.

It was Viagra that reopened the debate in 1998, followed by anti-obesity drugs and pointing the way to future developments of many new drugs with a spectrum of applications. These will range from 'medical necessity' through a 'medically useful but not essential' category to 'consumption for the purpose of personal gratification'.

Here, the authorities are staggering across a minefield littered with twisted logic. Most are denying the 'medical necessity' of such drugs altogether and refuse to reimburse them. Yet most of the conditions for which these drugs are being prescribed are, to say the least, health-damaging and often associated with actual disease. Total refusal to reimburse them may sound like acting on a principle but is clearly motivated by financial reasoning and ignores medical circumstances. That is one of the definitions of healthcare rationing.

Where the reimbursement rules discriminate between patients, as they do for Viagra in the UK, rationing is at work. No such distinctions are being applied to the general run of drugs which are normally prescribable in the NHS for *all approved indications*.

This area remains grey only because the definition of 'medical necessity' is shadowy. As precedents are set and more such drugs are introduced, it looks increasingly likely that decisions will cross the borderline into rationing. Such a move will suit centralised, public sector payers whose reimbursement decisions have no competitive motivation or objective.

iii) *Cash limits, volume restrictions and benefit caps*

Ostensibly, these are straightforward methods of cost containment, and mostly they work out as such. A grey area looms when these measures, or the penalties exacted for exceeding the limit are so harsh that they induce unsound medical decisions. These can take the form of shifting burdens between providers or changing treatments for *non-medical* reasons. For example, in-patients will become out-patients to balance the budget, or pharmaceutical prescribing is reduced in order to protect the physician's capped practice income. In their most obvious manifestation, cash limits create waiting lists, and rationing is in force.

iv) *Quality problems and below-standard outcomes*

The greater the pressure that is being applied to contain costs, the more likely is it that quality will be neglected or downgraded. The rising discontent of patients with American managed care is illustrative, although this discontent is fuelled more by anecdotal than by statistical evidence.

An opinion survey of 'non-institutionalised' adults in 1998 did indeed give 'traditional insurance' the edge over managed care on all published criteria, but the differences did not amount to wholesale condemnation of managed care. It was a matter of degree. Whereas only 23 per cent of those insured with traditional fee-for-service care considered that 'the healthcare system needs to be completely rebuilt', the corresponding response from those insured with managed care was 31 per cent. It was the *un*insured who, not surprisingly, gave a 59 per cent response.[4]

More generally, lack of compelling evidence of a serious quality crisis in health care, or of a proven link between cost containment and bad outcomes, are the main reasons for classifying these problems as a grey area.

Most interviews in preparation for this study led to expressions of doubt whether quality and outcome problems are to be laid at the door of cost containment and rationing, or are mainly attributable to weak and neglectful healthcare management. Wide disparities in providers' performance and outcomes for patients are common when comparing the results at different locations under the same healthcare system. Whilst rationing may be responsible for a proportion of these phenomena, a cause-and-effect link remains unproven.

v) *Level of complaints*

Again, complaints statistics give no clear lead on whether rationing is an important cause. Such complaints exist and are apt to balloon in media limelight, but these are the scandalous extremes. Little or nothing is known of the impact of rationing on the generality of complaints. It remains a grey area.

vi) *Absence of competition*

It is easier to *enforce* rationing in centralised *non*-competitive systems than under circumstances where market forces are allowed to operate. Rationing is also *less necessary* in competitive systems that can adjust more flexibly to changing circumstances and tend to regard rationing as uncompetitive and counter-productive.

On the other hand, it cannot be said that the lack of a competitive environment will unfailingly encourage rationing. The French healthcare system is probably the least competitively structured among major European nations, yet it is also the least rationed. Links between the absence of competition and healthcare rationing are grey-area questions.

vii) *'Invisible' rationing*

This was the expression used by several interviewees during discussions of healthcare rationing in Germany. 'Invisible' rationing is not overt but insidious: it creeps gradually into the healthcare system. Not decreed by law, it is nevertheless conditioned by the pressures arising from cost containment legislation.

Budgetary pressures, especially the threat of financial penalties in the event of excess spending will promote 'invisible' rationing. Among its manifestations are neglect of docile patients with little healthcare knowledge (neither inclined to answer back, nor capable of doing so), preferential treatment given to private patients, and using The Budget as an alibi for withholding or diluting treatment.

Elsewhere, the routine demand for pharmacoeconomic evidence as a *fourth hurdle* to reimbursement is a form of invisible rationing, because such evidence can be endlessly disputed among experts and used either to delay the reimbursement decision or to de-motivate doctors from prescribing. It is a characteristic grey-area tool.

The Symptoms And Tools Of Rationing

Passing from the grey area into the darkness of rationing, the following are noteworthy symptoms of the practice or tools of the trade:

i) Scarcity of physical resources

This remains one of the clearest causes of healthcare rationing. Doctors, nurses, facilities, equipment, or organs—some or all of these —may be in short supply. Rationing is not the only answer to shortages. Market responses would be to relieve the shortage as quickly as possible by all conceivable means and/or to raise incentives and, if necessary, prices.

In a centralised bureaucracy, however, rationing is administratively more convenient and conceptually more congenial than 'market' solutions. Moreover, in European health care, to raise prices in order to improve financial resources could run counter to the solidarity principle and would require a dose of political boldness that few governments would be willing to risk. Consequently, once shortages occur, they tend to persist and rationing will take root.

ii) Waiting lists and waiting times

These, too, are characteristic indicators of rationing unless waiting arises from purely temporary shortages. Long waiting lists or waiting times for elective surgery are a sure sign of a rationed healthcare system, because a shortage of physical resources makes delay in *non-*emergency operations more or less unavoidable.

iii) Denial of quality treatment

Under rationing, patients will be denied access to the best treatment in favour of cheaper alternatives. The main target of this type of rationing is innovation which carries a high price tag. Rationing will not be influenced by evidence demonstrating that innovative treatments will improve health outcomes, because rationing requires savings *now*, not in three, four or five years' time.

Rationing rather than normal cost containment is at work when the doctor's judgment is being overruled by a *non-*medical decision-maker, or when the system is procedurally skewed so as to propel the doctor in the desired direction regardless of medical preferences. When the pressure is significant but less extreme, the process moves back into the grey area of 'invisible' rationing.

iv) Discrimination between patients regardless of need

A fundamental principle of medicine is to treat patients in need. Rationing follows the same principle in theory but rarely in practice.

Criteria that are unrelated to need will find a place in the rulebook of rationing, because they help to make rationing 'bite'.

'Need' in health care is a concept that lacks precision. Most systems recognise need under conditions of emergency or when life is under threat. In chronic diseases, need is admitted more grudgingly. If a situation falls short of being medically compelling, need may be rebutted altogether. In rationing lingo, the word 'elective' sends a signal to administrators that the needs of rationing may be allowed to prevail over the patient's need. As rationing discriminates between patients, clinical need becomes subservient to financial constraint. Patients who need cheap treatments are not generally subjected to rationing. Cost becomes the arbiter of need.

This form of rationing 'regardless of need' can be extended *ad nauseam* to discriminate between patients on other than medical grounds. Among examples of this kind of discrimination are age, sex, lifestyle and place of residence.

'Ageism' relies upon spurious arguments for imposing age limits for certain interventions even though there is strong evidence that calendar age is not the main factor determining the success or failure of treatment. Indeed, increasing longevity is testimony to the effectiveness of most medical interventions, even for the 'oldest old' (85+) who are now the fastest growing segment of the population in the industrialised world. Ageism is a disguised form of rationing expenditure and discriminating in the use of scarce resources.

One of the more remarkable examples of sex discrimination was Japan's refusal even to register (let alone reimburse) oral contraceptives. Decades after their acceptance elsewhere in the industrialised world, the Japanese authorities eventually relented in 1999 when it began to look as though Viagra might actually reach the market ahead of the pill.

Ethics come into play when doctors judge a patient's lifestyle to be so reprehensible that they either threaten to withhold expensive forms of treatment or actually do so. Chain smokers who persistently refuse to stop or cut down but need costly operations or organ grafts exemplify the doctor's dilemma. Do they *deserve* expensive treatment and, if so, should they be relegated to the end of the waiting list? Here, rationing conspires with moral condemnation to ignore need. The recalcitrant smoker may not receive much public sympathy, but the principle is dangerous.

As technology advances, pressures to ration will become more intensive. A blatant disregard for need and its replacement by moral censure as the touchstone of discrimination between patients could place the medical profession in the invidious position of a 'health police'. Once we have condemned persistent smokers to death because we disapprove of their lack of will power, what is there to stop us from applying the same criteria to the obese (*let them lose weight*), the adventurous (*if you **will** climb Everest*), and the victims of sports injuries (*you expect **us** to pay for this boxer's traumatic brain injury?*). The blacklist could be extended indefinitely, to the HIV-positive, to drunken drivers, and to those deafened by lifelong addiction to fortissimo pop.

We should beware of letting the genie out of the bottle in the interests of rationing.

Finally, there is discrimination by place of residence—the notorious British practice known as 'postcode rationing'. It means that treatment may depend on demarcation lines between health authorities. One authority will pay, for example, for beta-interferon treatment of multiple sclerosis, another may refuse to do so. Treatment under the NHS then depends on where the patient lives. The practice is widely condemned, but the mindset of British healthcare policy was revealed by the reforms of 1999. Their aim is to do away with the postcode lottery by making rationing *fairer*, not by abolishing rationing.

4

When Rationing is Inevitable:
The Case of Organ Transplants

During the past 20 years, the grafting of organs has made spectacular strides technically. The development of immunosuppressive drugs to avert graft rejection, advances in transplantation technique, improvements in the storage and transport of organs to preserve their freshness, and substantial progress in tissue matching have all helped to establish organ transplantation as practicable and desirable.

Scarcity

There remains a central problem: a persistent and growing shortage of human organs. Transplantation operates in a world of scarcity. In the industrialised countries, scarcity—not money—is the most serious, sometimes fatal, obstacle. In all countries, including the market economy of the USA, the ability to pay is outlawed in guidelines for the selection of patients and the allocation of organs. Under conditions of genuine physical scarcity, one or other form of rationing is indeed inevitable.

Organ transplantation thus offers an unusual insight into the realities of healthcare rationing, and one that is largely uncontaminated by the finance factor. Cost-effectiveness can enter into the rules of selection and allocation. However, the clamour that 'we can't afford it' which is payers' standard response to costly forms of surgical or pharmaceutical intervention, is curiously muted in organ transplantation. Affordability is secondary when physical shortage dictates the volume of spending.

Waiting Lists

There are waiting lists (usually one of the prime symptoms of rationing) for most organs in all countries which supply statistics. In studying rationing, kidney grafts provide the most graphic example of shortage and of attempts to ration available supplies of donor organs.

This is shown in statistics published by Eurotransplant, an organisation that coordinates organ donation and allocation in several European countries. At the end of 1999, Austria, Belgium, Germany, Luxembourg and the Netherlands were members.

A mounting waiting list was made worse by the drop in cadaveric donations and fewer actual transplants. Many on the waiting list will die before they are called.

Table 1.4.1
Eurotransplant Waiting List for Organs, 31 December 1999

Organ	Waiting Patients	% Change from 31 December 1998
Kidney	12,131	+3
Pancreas	69	+11
Kidney + pancreas	193	+24
Heart	608	-15
Lung	345	+53
Heart + lung	46	-23

Source: Eurotransplant Foundation, press release 11 January 2000, www.transplant.org

The table points to the magnitude of the kidney shortage which is further illustrated by additional statistics:

Table 1.4.2
Cadaveric Kidney Donations and Transplants, 1999 (Eurotransplant Area)

	Number	% Change from 31 December 1998
Donations	2,446	-3
Transplants	2,766	-2

Source: Eurotransplant Foundation, press release 11 January 2000, www.transplant.org

In the United Kingdom, the waiting list for kidney grafts increased by 5.3 per cent in the 18 months between June 1998 and December 1999, from 4,526 to 4,767 (compare Germany: 9,217 at 31 December 1999, which was even worse). The problem in the UK is aggravated by another factor: while the waiting list is growing, 'the number of specialist surgeons available to carry out operations [is] shrinking,' according to the Royal College of Surgeons in England.[1] This professional shortage is a further—and, in the eyes of the profession, unnecessary—symptom of rationing.

In the USA, on 31 October 1998, the waiting list of the United Network for Organ Sharing (UNOS), a private contractor allocating organs on behalf of the Department of Health and Human Services, amounted to 63,994 persons. Of these, 66 per cent (41,576) were waiting for a kidney graft.[2] The kidney waiting list has risen rapidly and steadily from only about 27,000 in 1994.

Evidently, the shortage is widespread and unrelated to fundamental differences in healthcare systems. It arises primarily from a combination of rising demand with a relatively static organ supply.

Will The Shortage Of Supply Persist?

In the short and medium term, there is no way out of shortage. Longer term, the balance between supply and demand for some organs could be restored by xenotransplantation or organ regeneration using human embryonic tissue if these techniques are perfected and accepted by society. Xenotransplantation involves the grafting of animal organs into the human body. Technically, that will be feasible soon. Whether, and how quickly, society's fears about the risk of species-crossing infectious organisms, and reservations on ethical grounds, can be overcome, remains uncertain.

Meanwhile the main methods of alleviating organ shortage are to change the rules of *post mortem* ('cadaveric') organ donation, to encourage more living donors to come forward, and to improve organ management and the priorities of allocation.

At present, countries differ in their laws for the donation of cadaveric organs. Some require lifetime 'informed consent' by the deceased or *post mortem* family consent. Others lay down that organs shall be regarded as available for donation after death unless the deceased has formally opted out in his or her lifetime ('presumed consent').

Eurotransplant statistics demonstrate how 'presumed consent' can increase donation and help to alleviate the shortage of cadaveric organs. Austria, Belgium and Luxembourg operate a 'presumed consent' system, whereas Germany and the Netherlands require 'informed consent'.

The 'presumed consent' system has produced about double the number of donors per head of population when compared with the 'informed consent' rules. There is a similar relationship in the number of transplants *per capita*. Consequently, in 1999, the waiting list for kidney transplants fell by nine per cent in Austria and by 13 per cent in Belgium, whereas it rose by four per cent in Germany and by 12 per cent in the Netherlands. However, sizeable waiting lists remained in all countries.

Table 1.4.3

Transplants and cadaveric donors per million population, 1999

Country	Consent	Transplants	Donors
Austria	presumed	87	25
Belgium/Lux	presumed	70	23
Germany	informed	41	12
Netherlands	informed	31	10

Source: Eurotransplant Foundation, press release 11 January 2000,
www.transplant.org

The use of grafts is rationed either formally or informally. The formal process will be governed by rules and guidelines for transplant centres. Informal rationing may leave more room for manoeuvre and the exercise of discretion at local level.

Three principal rationing decisions determine the patient's chance of obtaining an organ graft:

i)   Admittance to the waiting list

ii)   Allocation of an available tissue-matched organ

iii)   Decision to implant an allocated organ in a waiting patient

Collectively, these decisions conform to the classic concept of health-care rationing, involving discrimination between patients under conditions of scarcity. The first determines whether a patient is to be regarded as eligible for a transplant. If not, entry to the waiting list is barred. The second considers to whom, among numerous waiting and tissue-matched patients of (theoretically) equal merit and urgency, a newly available organ should be allocated. The third decision, although a logical consequence of the first two, can be upset or reversed by unforeseen emergencies affecting patients or organs. The designated patient may not be fit enough when the organ arrives (the majority of transplant patients have serious co-morbidities), or the organ may arrive too late or in bad condition. One does not queue for organs as one might for tickets to hear the Three Tenors.

Allocation Of Organs

Rationing kidney grafts is complicated by the fact that, in contrast to other organs, there is an alternative: end-stage renal dialysis (ESRD).

However, ESRD facilities are also stretched or even rationed, and dialysis is ultimately more expensive than transplantation because it is for life. Many patients dislike the inconvenience and persistence of ESRD which can prevent them from leading normal lives.

The problem of allocating kidney grafts in the USA has been trenchantly described:

> This frequently rancorous debate has pitted patient against patient, physician against physician, smaller hospitals against larger institutions, and politicians from states with large multiorgan-transplantation programs against those from states with smaller programs.[3]

In the USA, in 1996, an estimated 93 per cent of ESRD patients were covered by Medicare, the federal programme for seniors and certain groups of disabled patients. The number of ESRD patients had nearly quadrupled from 48,000 in 1978 to 188,000 in 1996. By the end of that year, 75 per cent of patients were on dialysis and 25 per cent had functioning kidney grafts. The proportion of graft carriers (which had been only 13.5 per cent in 1978) fell slightly during the first half of the 1990s because of the organ shortage:

> The slowing of the rate of increase in functioning graft beneficiaries is unfortunate since they have a better quality of life and their expenditures for medical care are much lower than dialysis patients.[4]

In other words, not only do kidney grafts have to be rationed, but their scarcity also impedes the progress of containing the cost of dialysis and leaves patients at a medical and lifestyle disadvantage.

The existing system of organ allocation in the USA is geographical. The waiting lists of the nearest transplant centres come first, then regional centres, finally national distribution. The situation raises curious echoes of the notorious postcode rationing practice in the UK. Indeed, the US Department of Health and Human Services (DHHS) proposed revised regulations in October 1999 that 'would direct organs to the sickest patients first, regardless of where they live'.[5]

A 'sickest patients first' policy sounds reassuringly fair but is not necessarily the most practical solution when perishable organs are being allocated across a continental area. A study based on simulated models has examined four alternative 'allocation policies for rationing kidneys among blood group-compatible candidates on the local transplant waiting list', namely:

1. First-come-first-transplanted

2. Point system used by UNOS (based on points for waiting time, rank in waiting list, degree of tissue-matching, etc)

3. Efficiency-based allocation to maximise Quality-Adjusted Life Expectancy (QALE)

4. 'Distributive efficiency' which aims additionally to reduce race, sex and age discrimination in organ allocation

The study's aim was to address the organ shortage by investigating how the effectiveness of allocation could be improved, because neither of the two main alternatives are as yet practicable: improving supply by adopting 'presumed consent' (which remains illegal in the USA), or major technical advances in transplantation.

The study concluded that a 'sickest patients first' policy 'where an alternative therapy, dialysis, is available' would actually be counter-productive. It would result 'in an *increase* in overall waiting times and lower patient and graft survival'. It advocated the 'distributive efficiency' model whose adoption, it estimated, would be equivalent to what 'would be achieved by a 23 per cent increase in the supply of donor organs'.[6]

Selection Of Patients

The above-mentioned study shows that the interaction of cause and effect in healthcare rationing under conditions of physical scarcity is much more complex than common-sense concepts of rationing would suggest. In the example cited above, the proposed solution is in effect counter-intuitive. This points to the need for caution when policy makers interpret the results of opinion surveys on the subject of healthcare rationing, because respondents may rely largely on common sense and the promptings of emotional triggers.

This is illustrated by a British survey of public opinion and of clinicians on the priorities of patient selection for donor liver grafts. There are no official guidelines for patient selection for organ transplants in the UK.

Given eight hypothetical case histories, respondents (the public, family doctors and gastroenterologists) were asked to pick four out of seven preferred allocation criteria from among the following:

1. time on waiting list
2. age
3. value of patient to society
4. alcohol consumption (related to liver disease)
5. work status
6. outcome of transplant in terms of life expectancy
7. drug abuse (related to liver disease).

There was a clear variation in priorities between the three groups. While the general public thought that priority should be given to younger children, those with a better outcome, and those who had waited longest, the gastroenterologists gave high priority to outcome alone. The family doctors put priorities intermediate between the two other groups.[7]

The survey revealed a gulf between the professionals and the public's relatively emotional approach to patient selection, though even the public made the outcome criterion its second choice. For the professionals, outcome was paramount but even among them there was no lack of emotional response: when prioritising four of the eight hypothetical patients, rejection by the professionals of the prisoner and the man with alcoholic liver disease was almost as absolute as that of the general public. The authors contrast these findings with the American Medical Association's selection rules for organ grafts which list five *unacceptable* criteria:

> Ability to pay, contribution of the patient to society, perceived obstacles to treatment (such as alcohol abuse ...), the contribution of the patient to his or her medical condition (...) and past use of medical resources.[8]

The inference from the results of the survey is that 'real life' health-care rationing will be tinged up to a point by the core emotions of the individual professional decision maker. Official guidelines will help to make more rational choices, but in practice they will not be applied to every patient. Even specialists will draw the line at some patients, whatever the guidelines say. Yet moral censure, ageism (quite strongly in evidence in the responses to Neuberger *et al*'s survey), and other modes of personal preference or prejudice are damaging and need to be repressed.

The case of organ grafts shows how difficult it is to ration health care rationally, equitably and effectively, even when conditions of physical scarcity make rationing 'inevitable'. There is confusion between the slogans of politicians and factual evidence which may be counter-intuitive. There is a gulf between what sounds good and what will actually work. There is a rift between the desires of the general public and the professional judgment of transplantation specialists. Finally, closer to the operating theatre, there are the problems of day-to-day management of scarcity while organs and patients fail to conform to the rules laid down in textbooks.

If that is the situation where there is no workable alternative option, it would seem that rationing should be shunned whenever it is avoidable. Part II of this study compares international experience and probes the question why some countries seem to be avoiding what others regard as inevitable.

Part II

International Comparisons

We might have less of a rationing problem if we spent a little more on health.

John Grimley Evans, 1997

International comparisons are rarely based on precisely comparable statistics. Countries vary in their definitions of 'health care' and data can be changed prospectively and retrospectively if terms are re-defined or reviewed. Often, the same parameters are reported with quite different numbers in a variety of sources. In this study, the difficulty of accurately comparing health data between countries is addressed in two ways:

i) Whenever possible, the health database of the Organisation for Economic Cooperation and Development (OECD) has been used. This, more than most sources, is the result of deliberate efforts to achieve comparability between countries. Even the OECD, how-ever, is far from claiming perfection in this respect.

ii) A relatively large number of parameters of comparison are used, if available, as a basis for drawing broad conclusions.

1

Health Expenditure and Resources

Total Healthcare Expenditure As A Percentage of Gross Domestic Product (GDP)

This is probably the most widely used measure for comparing the allocation of wealth to health. The commonly accepted view is that wealthier nations can afford to spend more on health and do so. This correlation is broadly proven but is not precise, because other factors also influence the intensity of healthcare spending, for example: willingness to spend, control systems, efficiency, political priorities, and healthcare 'culture'.

For the years 1980, 1990, 1998 and 1999, the countries covered by this study compare with one another and with the OECD median ratio as follows:

Table 2.1.1
Total Healthcare Expenditure, Percentage of GDP

Country	1980	1990	1998	1999	% change 1980-1999
UK	5.7	6.0	6.7	7.0	+23
France	7.4	8.8	9.6	9.5	+28
Germany	8.8	8.7	10.6	10.5	+19
USA	8.9	12.4	13.6	13.7	+54
OECD median	6.7	7.2	7.6*		+13*

Note: * 1997 (medians not yet available for 1998,1999)
Source: *OECD Health Data 2000*; medians—author's calculation.
　　　　1980: 26 countries; 1990, 1997: 29 countries

Among the four listed countries, the UK spent the lowest proportion of GDP on health throughout the period, although it participated in the rising trend. The gap between the UK and France/Germany was nevertheless much higher than one would normally expect of economically similar European countries. In 1999, the ratio for the UK was 26 per cent below that for France and 33 per cent below Germany's. It was just over half the US ratio and lower even than the 1997 median of the 29 member states of the OECD which includes three Eastern European states and three developing countries.

Separate analysis of public and private health expenditure gives the following picture:

Table 2.1.2
Public Healthcare Expenditure, Percentage of GDP

Country	1980	1998	1999	% change 1980-1999	OECD rank 1998
UK	5.1	5.6	5.9	+16	18
France	5.8	7.3	7.3	+26	5
Germany	6.9	7.9	7.9	+14	1
USA	3.7	6.1	6.1	+65	12
OECD median (1997)		5.9		+13	

Source: *OECD Health Data 2000*; medians—author's calculation.
1980: 26 countries; 1990, 1997: 29 countries

The UK's position is similar to that for total health expenditure, but the gaps are somewhat narrower: the UK's public expenditure ratio is 19 per cent lower than France's, 25 per cent below Germany's, and three per cent lower even than the *public* expenditure ratio of the USA. Indeed, the USA in 1998 ranked 12th among the 29 OECD member states in the proportion of GDP spent on *public* health care. Its transformation from its position in 1980 is possibly the most important change in the funding of health care in the industrialised world during the past 20 years.

Table 2.1.3
Private Healthcare Expenditure, Percentage of GDP

Country	1980	1998	1999	% change 1980-1999	OECD rank 1998
UK	0.6	1.1	1.1	+83	25
France	1.6	2.3	2.2	+38	12
Germany	1.9	2.7	2.6	+37	3
USA	5.2	7.5	7.6	+46	1
OECD median (1997)		1.8			

Source: *OECD Health Data 2000*; median—author's calculation.
1980: 26 countries; 1990, 1997: 29 countries

Table 2.1.3 demonstrates the abnormally low proportion of GDP spent on *private* health care in the UK. Although the ratio has grown faster than that of France and Germany, it was still some 50-60 per cent lower than in both these countries in 1999. The British ratio was far below the OECD median, ranking the UK 25th out of 29 in 1998 —an altogether extraordinary situation.

The pre-eminent position of the USA in the proportion of GDP spent on private health care is no surprise. Contrary to the US trend in public spending, however, the private ratio has been essentially static since 1990 when it was already 7.5 per cent.

The Significance Of Healthcare/GDP Ratios

This ratio will be affected by changes both in the numerator (health expenditure) and in the denominator (GDP). It will rise if healthcare spending increases faster than GDP, for example in periods of recession, and can fall at times of rapid economic growth.

The 'normal' trend over the last four decades has been a rise in the proportion of GDP devoted to health care. The *income elasticity* of healthcare spending has been estimated as about 1.3 (±0.1) for the then 12 member states of the European Union between 1974 and 1994,[1] and 1.5 for the USA over the period 1980-1992.[2] In other words, for every percentage point of change in GDP, health expenditure was observed to have changed by 1.3 and 1.5 percentage points, respectively.

The income elasticity of health expenditure may have fallen during the second half of the 1990s, a period of rapid economic growth in the USA and UK, and more intensive cost containment of health care everywhere. This was not unprecedented. For example, between 1990 and 1998, both total and public expenditure on health declined in Sweden and Finland, and the *public* ratio also fell significantly in Canada, Denmark and Italy. Most other countries were either stable or their healthcare spending continued to rise faster than their GDP. Even in the USA, however, the *total* expenditure ratio fell by 0.4 points and the public ratio by 0.4 points between 1995 and 1999 as economic growth quickened and healthcare cost containment became tougher under managed care.

Widely expressed fears that healthcare spending is growing *uncontrollably*, to the point where health will ultimately devour wealth, make good headlines but little sense. They are based on the extrapolation of past trends *ad absurdum*. Serious danger would arise only during periods of severe economic depression. At such times, it would prove difficult to throttle back health spending in the ageing societies of the industrialised world.

Health Expenditure Per Head Of Population

Another way of comparing spending on health care is per head of population. When measuring this in US dollars, the impact of fluctuating exchange rates can be reduced by using purchasing power parities ($PPP) which are adjusted for differences in the cost of living. Since OECD uses a general basket of goods and services for calculating $PPPs (not a healthcare basket), national differences in healthcare prices are not entirely eliminated. For the countries compared here, $PPP in place of exchange rate $ widens the difference between US and European *per capita* health expenditures in recent years but narrows that between the UK and France/Germany.

Health expenditure per head of population is less directly affected by GDP than the preceding statistics and linked more closely with what each nation is willing to spend on health care. This is brought out clearly in the following table:

Table 2.1.4
Healthcare Expenditure Per Head of Population,
1999 ($PPP)

Country	Total	Public	Private
UK	1,583	1,333	250
France	2,130	1,631	499
Germany	2,476	1,863	613
USA	4,390	1,942	2,448

Source: *OECD Health Data 2000*

The UK spends far less on total health care per head of population than the three other countries: 26 per cent less than France, 36 per cent less than Germany, and roughly one-third of the American level.

For public expenditure, the USA actually spends more per head than any of the three European countries, but this is probably attributable mainly to high prices. Even in public expenditure *per capita*, the UK lags seriously behind France (by 18 per cent) and Germany (by 28 per cent).

The most striking differences, however, are those in private health-care spending per head of population. Here, UK spending is half of that in France and two-fifths of the German level. Whereas in the latter countries, private expenditure is approximately one-quarter of total spending, in the UK the private share is less than one-sixth.

The UK situation cannot be explained by relative 'poverty'. In 1999, GDP *per capita* in $PPP compared as follows:

Table 2.1.5
Gross Domestic Product Per Head of Population

	GDP in $PPP
UK	22,459
France	22,465
Germany	23,616
USA	31,935

Source: *OECD Health Data 2000*

The UK's GDP per head of population was the same as in France and only 4.9 per cent below Germany's. These narrow differentials cannot adequately explain the wide disparities in *per capita* spending in terms of 'income elasticity'. Other factors like lack of political will to spend more on health care or to encourage an upsurge of private spending, as well as cultural differences, including medical culture, are probably more potent influences on low UK spending than incomes.

The spending pattern of the UK diverges to an extraordinary degree from those of France, Germany and the USA. Its *per capita* expenditure on health care ranks low in the spectrum of all 29 OECD member states.

Table 2.1.6
Ranking Order of Per Capita Expenditure on Health Care, 1998, OECD member states, Rank out of 29 by value $PPP

Country	Total	Public	Private
UK	18	16	22
France	10	10	10
Germany	4	6	5
USA	1	4	1

Source: *OECD Health Data 2000*

Rich countries have options. They can either spend prolifically per head of population on both public and private health care, like the USA (ranked 4th and 1st, respectively) and Switzerland (ranked 1st and 2nd). Alternatively, the public purse can spend on a lavish scale and make private spending unnecessary, as in Luxembourg (ranked 2nd for public and 23rd for private spending). The emphasis can also be shifted towards private spending, as in the Netherlands (ranked 12th and 6[th,] respectively).

The position of the UK in the *per capita* ranks (public 16th and private 22nd) is almost incomprehensible. It is anomalous in relation to the country's economic status; so much so that one needs to look for an explanation in *political*, not in economic or financial, terms. Either the policies of successive governments, or the popular will, or an amalgam of the two, have consistently kept public expenditure per head of the British population low, and discouraged private spending. Already in 1980, the UK's rank for total *per capita* healthcare expenditure was 20th out of 25, wedged between Ireland and Greece. By 1998, the UK had risen to 18th out of 29. Big deal.

It is the picture of a rich country in which health care is rationed.

Component Elements Of Healthcare Expenditure Per Capita ($PPP)

The results are broadly the same when *per capita* spending on hospitals, physicians and pharmaceuticals is analysed separately. Among OECD member states in 1996, the UK ranked 18th out of 29 for hospital expenditure per head of population, 14th out of 20 for physician services, and 17th out of 25 for pharmaceuticals.[3]

Resources

The number of physicians per 1,000 population in 1998 was recorded as follows:

Table 2.1.7
Number of Practising Physicians Per 1,000 Population, 1998

UK	1.7
France	3.0
Germany	3.5
USA	2.7
OECD (median 1996)	2.8

Source: *OECD Health Data 2000*

France and Germany acknowledge that they have a surplus of doctors and are trying to reduce this by discouraging entry into the profession. The UK is at the other end of the scale, with a considerable shortage. The UK ranks 26th out of 29 OECD member states. Only Mexico, South Korea and Turkey have fewer physicians per 1,000 population.

The situation for nurses shows similar deficits in the UK compared with France, Germany and the USA:

Table 2.1.8
Number of Practising Certified Registered Nurses
Per 1,000 Population, 1998

UK	5.0
France	5.9*
Germany	9.6
USA	8.3

Note: * 1997
Source: *OECD Health Data 2000*

Among OECD member states, only Greece, South Korea, Mexico, Portugal and Turkey have fewer registered nurses per 1,000 population than the UK.

By contrast with the meagre level of its healthcare resources, the UK is relatively efficient in their use. Physician consultations *per capita* compare as follows:

Table 2.1.9
Physician Consultations Per Capita, 1996

UK	6.1
France	6.5
Germany	6.5
USA	5.8
OECD median	5.9

Source: *OECD Health Data 2000*

Here the UK was just above the OECD median and close to the three other countries in 1996, although UK consultations fell to 5.4 in 1998 (no comparable figures for 1998 are available for the other three countries).

What these statistics do not reveal is the length and quality of the average consultation. With a much lower physician density and a similar number of consultations per head of population, UK patients will be given less time by their doctors than those in the other three countries. (For the USA, this is confirmed in a survey of British and American patients in Part II-3).

The UK's relatively strong performance when compared with France and Germany also shows up in efficiency ratios for hospitals: beds per 1,000 people, hospital days *per capita*, and average length of stay per patient. In all these, the UK pattern resembles that of the USA.

Unfortunately, efficiency in health care can go too far. There comes a point when utilisation is so intensive that resources become depleted, either creating shortages or achieving productivity at the expense of quality. Whereas American managed care is accused of the latter, the NHS is clearly experiencing both.

Conclusions

During the past 20 years, the United Kingdom has consistently spent far less on health care as a percentage of Gross Domestic Product and per head of population than France and Germany (countries with comparable national income per head of population) and the USA.

The gap between the UK and the other three countries applies to public as well as private expenditure on health, but is extraordinarily wide for the latter. Indeed, private expenditure on health in the UK is *abnormally* low by international standards, ranking 25th out of 29 OECD member states as percentage of GDP and 22nd out of 29 per head of population.

As a concomitant of its low overall level of public and private spending on health, the UK is seriously under-resourced in terms of doctors and nurses: per head of population, it ranks respectively 26th and 24th out of 29 OECD member states. In some of these ratios, the UK is closer in the ranking order to Mexico, South Korea and Turkey than it is to France, Germany and the USA.

On the other hand, the UK's productivity ratios in health care are similar to those of France, Germany and the USA, suggesting that efficiency in the use of resources is at least comparable. Whether under-resourcing has affected health outcomes is examined in the following chapter.

2

Morbidity and Outcomes

The relative efficiency of the NHS in using its very limited resources is widely recognised. The official line of successive governments has been to stress that the NHS is not only efficient but also effective. The argument goes that the UK spends less but scores no worse than comparable countries (who spend much more) in comparisons of commonly accepted indicators of health status, such as life expectancy and infant mortality.

This view and the parameters on which it is based should be challenged. Neither of the two indicators is a realistic criterion of the effectiveness of health care in the industrialised countries at the beginning of the twenty-first century.

Both indicators represent problems that were extremely grave in the nineteenth century and still serious in the first half of the twentieth. By the late decades of the last century, both were well past their crisis points. By 1996, the outliers among OECD member states for infant mortality per 1,000 live births were Hungary 10.6, Poland 12.3, Mexico 17.0 and Turkey 42.2, compared with the UK 6.2 and the OECD median 5.8.[1] Moreover, it is unclear to what extent the reductions in infant mortality and the extensions of life expectancy are due specifically to better health care as distinct from a combination of factors including advances in public health and sanitation, as well as education and personal hygiene. To suggest that life expectancy and infant mortality statistics constitute an alibi for the effectiveness of the NHS verges on the eccentric.

Effective health care in rich countries today is above all a question of the control of morbidity. We live longer, not necessarily healthier lives. Morbidity from stress, mental imbalances, asthma, malignancies and many other conditions is rising, and longer life expectancy has brought the problem of chronic diseases into greater prominence than in the past. Modern health care will be increasingly involved in prevention, innovative surgery and pharmaceuticals, gene therapy, the quality of patients' lives, and long-term care as those who survive into the highest age groups become frail and physically dependent.

The effectiveness of health care for the elderly segment of the population can be partially represented by life expectancy *at age 65*, although even this is still a measure of mortality, not of health status in old age.

Table 2.2.1
Life Expectancy at Age 65 (1996)
(years)

	Female	Male
UK	18.4	14.7
France	20.6	16.1
Germany	18.6	14.9
USA	18.9	15.7

Source: Anderson and Poullier, 'Health spending, access and outcomes', 1999.

The UK and Germany show up less well than the USA and especially France. The British and German figures are also below the OECD median. The highest life expectancy at 65 was recorded in Japan for both females (21.5) and males (16.9). Again, the interplay of a variety of causes in producing these results are not clear. Is health care a more important influence in determining life expectancy at 65 than life-styles, genetics, social support, or poverty?

Two other approaches, still based on mortality because comparable morbidity statistics are not available, compare the four countries in terms of their mortality rates at different ages and by the principal causes of death.

Table 2.2.2
Death Rates Per 100,000 Population: All Ages, All Causes

	Female	Male
UK	1,121	1,082
France	839	960
Germany	1,130	1,034
USA	838	915

Source: *World Health Statistics 1996*, WHO 1998.

France and the USA have considerably lower death rates from all causes than the UK and Germany. France, as noted above, has higher life expectancy at age 65 (after which most deaths occur), whereas the USA is demographically younger. This would imply lower death rates, other things being equal. Further analysis of death rates from all causes per 100,000 of various age groups in each of the four countries indicates that:

At age 45-54: UK death rates are the lowest for males and more or less in line with France and Germany for females. The USA has the highest death rates.

At age 55-64: Basically a similar pattern as for 45-54, although the relative position of the UK *vis-à-vis* France and Germany is worsening.

At age 65-74: For this age group, the UK has the highest death rates for both females and males. The relative position of the USA shows a marked improvement, whilst France stands out with by far the lowest death rates for both sexes.

At age 75+: The USA emerges with the lowest death rates per 100,000 for males, and effectively on a par with France for females. The UK and Germany record much higher rates for both sexes.

Table 2.2.3
Causes of Death: All Ages
(rates per 100,000 population)

Circulatory Causes

	Female	Male
UK	485	462
France	305	273
Germany	598	449
USA	372	353

Cancers

	Female	Male
UK	253	287
France	186	304
Germany	249	273
USA	191	221

Respiratory causes

	Female	Male
UK	185	160
France	60	69
Germany	61	73
USA	79	83

Source: *World Health Statistics 1996*, WHO 1998.

The analysis suggests (though it does not prove) that, in the UK, weaknesses in health care for the over-65 age group may be partially responsible for higher overall mortality rates than in France and the USA. This applies particularly to the 65-74 age group but also to the 75+ segment.

UK death rates for the two younger age groups show up well by comparison with the other countries and suggest that healthcare performance for the age range 45-64 in the UK is adequate or better.

France has the lowest death rates from all three of the above causes, except for cancer in males. The USA has a good record in circulatory and respiratory mortality rates. Germany has high death rates for circulatory causes (especially female) and cancers but is broadly in line with France for respiratory causes.

The UK has the highest death rates for circulatory causes (male), cancers (females), and abnormally high mortality from respiratory diseases for both sexes.

Two major causes of death where mortality rates in the UK are far higher than for any of the other three countries are breast cancer and pneumonia.

Table 2.2.4
Death Rates from Breast Cancer Per 100,000 Population, by Age Group

Age	45-64	55-64	65-74	75+
UK	53	85	120	201
France	40	71	93	161
Germany	48	74	105	179
USA	42	70	106	160

Source: *World Health Statistics 1996*, WHO 1998.

Death rates from breast cancer in the UK are at least 15-20 per cent higher than in the three other countries. France (especially for the 64-75s) and the USA have the lowest rates.

Table 2.2.5
Death Rates from Pneumonia per 100,000 Population by Age Group

Age	55-64		65-74		75+	
	Male	Female	Male	Female	Male	Female
UK	33	22	153	106	1,304	1,233
France	15	5	45	17	415	296
Germany	11	4	43	20	345	237
USA	21	12	74	42	492	385

Source: *World Health Statistics 1996*, WHO 1998.

UK death rates from pneumonia, already excessive at age 55-64, escalate rapidly after the age of 65. Although escalation with rising age occurs everywhere, the death rate from pneumonia for the over-75s towers above those for France, Germany and the USA. Unless there is mis-reporting of the cause of death on a massive scale, there must be grounds for attributing the abnormally high incidence of UK deaths from pneumonia—a disease that is often preventable and curable—to neglect of the very old and to cross-infection in hospitals.

Not all mortality statistics for major causes of death show the UK in an unfavourable light. When compared with France (the 'gold standard'), death rates are similar for colon cancer, prostate cancer, leukaemia, diabetes and kidney diseases. They are lower in the UK for liver diseases. However, one has to comb through the statistics with diligence and persistence to find major causes of death for which British levels per 100,000 population are as low as in France, or lower.

UK standards of care in the 'killer' diseases (heart and cancer) are also reported to be below those of the USA and most of Europe. The UK is slow to adopt innovative pharmaceuticals, diagnostics, surgical interventions and methods of after-care. Outcomes in terms of five-year rates of survival after treatment are generally poor. Specialist skills are excellent but in short supply. A review of the two disease areas has concluded (on cancer) that: 'Some of the disparities were due to bad or inconsistent clinical practice, but the underlying difficulty was the lack of finance'. The overall conclusion was that 'there is little doubt that rationing is the root cause of these problems'.[2]

3

Satisfaction and Opinion Surveys

There is no such a thing as a free lunch—or is there?

The Trouble With Surveys

Opinion surveys are a matter of opinion. 'Satisfaction' is an indicator of how the general public perceives the functioning of its healthcare system. It is an important but treacherous form of guidance for politicians and reformers. Politicians believe that opinion polls will help them to gauge electoral sentiment. Reformers (in government, opposition, and pressure groups) want to know whether their efforts are likely to have a 'following wind' or whether the public is satisfied with the existing healthcare system and indifferent to reform.

The interpretation of satisfaction and opinion surveys in health care is not easy. Much depends on how the questions are phrased and the emotional temperature of their wording. Some questions will lead to a predictable majority of politically correct answers.

In the UK, for example, the answer to the question *'Should the government be spending more on the NHS?'* will always be an overwhelming 'YES'. Even when the question is refined (as in an actual British Social Attitudes survey of 1998) by adding the words 'even if this means an increase in tax?', the answer is a fairly predictable majority in favour (68 per cent).

That Is The Trap Of The 'Hypothetical Purchase'

Respondents are only *hypothetically* paying more tax for more health care. They are not (yet) being asked to pay up with real additional deductions from their personal disposable incomes.

To predict how opinion surveys that contain hypothetical purchase propositions will translate into real-life electoral support is like walking across a row of trap doors in the dark. You cannot tell whether they are open or shut.

Trends in satisfaction and opinion surveys are equally problematic. A report by the UK Royal Commission on Long-Term Care has drawn a distinction between *period effects, life-cycle effects*, and *generational effects* when analysing age cohorts. A *period effect* is the result of external conditions at or near the time of the survey. A *life-cycle effect* observes 'changes that occur as people get older', whilst a *generational*

50

effect is related to the respondent's year of birth and typical 'of a *particular* group brought up in a *particular* era' which may colour their attitudes for the rest of their lives.[1]

Most published reports of attitudes and trends fall short of these sophisticated forms of analysis and presentation, and can give only a crude impression of the state or trend of public opinion. In the following international comparisons, the four countries covered by this study have been extracted from survey results that may have included other countries. The latter are shown only where this is thought illuminating.

On The Public's Satisfaction With The Healthcare System 'In Our Country' (1996)

Respondents in member states of the European Union (EU) were asked whether they were satisfied (on a five-point scale: very/fairly satisfied, neither satisfied nor dissatisfied, fairly/very dissatisfied) with the healthcare system in their country. Disregarding the 'neither/nor' respondents and those classified as 'other', the following results were obtained:

Table 2.3.1
Satisfaction with Healthcare System 'In Our Country'

	% Satisfied ('very' or 'fairly')	% Dissatisfied ('very' or 'fairly')	Difference ± % points
UK	48.1	40.9	+7.2
France	65.1	14.6	+50.5
Germany	66.0	10.9	+55.1

Source: Mossialos, E., 1997.[2]

The survey showed a high degree of public satisfaction with the healthcare systems in France and Germany, and a barely positive view in the UK. The only countries where dissatisfaction exceeded satisfaction were Greece (-35.5), Portugal (-39.4) and Italy (-43.1). Denmark produced the most positive response (+ 80.4).

The UK response may have been affected unfavourably by the *period effect* in 1996. British Social Attitudes has observed 'rising satisfaction when extra funds are spent on the health service ... higher level of dissatisfaction (indeed the highest ever) in 1996 when no extra money was made available for the NHS'.[3] In fact, the British Social Attitudes survey produced worse results in 1996 than Mossialos: only 36 per cent satisfaction compared with 50 per cent dissatisfaction (net -14 per cent). This may have been caused by sampling differences or by a slight variance in the way in which the question was phrased.

In a variant of seeking opinions on 'the way health care is run in [our country]', British Social Attitudes asked about 'the way in which the National Health Service is run nowadays'. The substitution of the NHS for 'health care' may have induced respondents to think more politically and less about health care received from 'my own doctor'. Also the word 'nowadays' is less neutral than 'in our country'. 'Nowadays' could evoke contrarian echoes of 'the good old days'. That is, of course, pure supposition, but the different results of the two surveys in the same year suggest that the conclusions to be drawn from opinion surveys are best kept very broad.

Very broadly then, the French and the Germans were more satisfied with their healthcare system in 1996 than the British. Events since then may well have reduced the level of satisfaction in all three countries but are unlikely to have moved in favour of the UK.

On The Need For 'Fundamental Changes'

The last published comprehensive comparison of the countries covered by the present study relates to the years 1988-1991 and is not necessarily a reliable indicator of attitudes towards healthcare reform today. The question was whether respondents consider that 'only minor changes are necessary' or that 'fundamental changes are needed' or even that 'we need to completely rebuild' the system. Adding up the 'fundamental changes' and 'rebuild' responses gave the following picture:

Table 2.3.2
Survey Responses 1988-1991
'Fundamentally change/rebuild' the healthcare system

	%
UK	69
France	52
Germany	48
USA	89

Sources: various, quoted in *OECD Health Data 99*.[4]

As was the case with the 'satisfaction' survey of 1996, France and Germany appeared at least half-contented with their existing healthcare system whereas more than two-thirds of the British sample wanted fundamental changes. In the USA, there was an overwhelming desire for reform, with 29 per cent actually wanting 'complete rebuilding' of the system. However, the *hypothetical purchase* trap was well and truly sprung in the USA. Only a few years later, President Clinton's reform plan, which involved *very* fundamental changes, collapsed in a welter of political controversy and without much protest from the general public.

By 1994, the year when the Clinton plan became a heap of ashes, a further comparison between the USA and Germany still showed 81 per cent of Americans in favour of 'fundamental changes' or rebuilding, compared with 66 per cent in Germany[5] where there had been a strong swing against the existing system.

Direct comparison between the UK and the USA was reported for 1998 when the desire for fundamental reform and rebuilding in the USA had sagged a little further, to a still handsome majority of 77 per cent, whilst that in the UK had remained relatively static: 72 per cent compared with 69 per cent in 1990.[6] Considering that the UK had been through a major and in some respects fundamental healthcare reform under Margaret Thatcher in 1990, and that further reforms were announced by the Blair government in 1998, the public's insatiable appetite for reform looks more apparent than real.

Reformers would be ill-advised to interpret these survey responses as genuine pressure for fundamental reform. They are more likely to represent characteristic British grumbling to the effect that *'they* (politicians) should really do something about health care.'

Meanwhile, the Mossialos survey had also shown the public's theoretical longing for reform as greater than its 'dissatisfaction'. Omitting those who said that only minor changes are needed, views about the existing healthcare system in 1996 were as follows:

Table 2.3.3
European Survey Responses 1996
(Views about the country's healthcare system)

Dissatisfied	Country	'Runs quite well'	Fundamentally change/rebuild	Difference ± % points
		%	%	%
40.9	UK	14.6	56.0	-41.4
14.6	France	25.6	29.6	-4.0
10.9	Germany	36.9	18.9	+18.0

Source: Mossialos, 1997.[7]

By 1996, Germany had experienced a succession of moderately fundamental health reforms since 1979 and the public had evidently had enough. In France, opinion was balanced, with a slight (possibly insignificant) bias in favour of reform. With low levels of dissatisfaction and a history of gradual rather than radical reforms during the preceding decade, France basically supported the *status quo*. The UK again displayed far more desire for fundamental change (though less so than in the survey by Donelan, Blendon *et al* of 1998, see above), but the *grumble hypothesis* was probably in action here, too.

The 'Grumble Hypothesis'

The clue to the British situation is the difference between a general and not unhealthy tendency to grumble and let off steam, and a remarkably low level of protest about the treatment that individual respondents and their families have actually received on the NHS.

Donelan, Blendon *et al.*,[8] compared responses of 'non-institutionalised' adults in five markets including the UK and the USA. The following views of respondents' *personal* experience compare the combined answers 'excellent' and 'very good' with the combined responses 'fair' and 'poor':

Table 2.3.4
Personal Experience of Medical Care, 1998

Question	Country	Excellent + very good %	Fair + Poor %	Difference ± % points
Medical care received by self + family in past year	UK	50	14	+36
	USA	49	15	+34
Care received at last doctor visit	UK	56	14	+42
	USA	59	16	+43
Overall experience of hospital care	UK	62	18	+44
	USA	54	18	+36

Source: Donelan, Blendon *et al.*[9]

These very positive responses contradict the degree of dissatisfaction expressed about the system in general. They are also curiously at variance with the insistent yearning for 'fundamental' reform and total 'rebuilding'. For the UK, this seems to confirm the potency of the grumble hypothesis in satisfaction surveys.

On the other hand, even when British respondents have something tangible to grumble about, they are quite reluctant to spit it out:

Table 2.3.5
Further Personal Experience of Medical Care, 1998

Question	Country	%	Under 10 minutes %	Over 15 minutes %
Length of time of the most recent doctor visit	UK		65	12
	USA		30	48
Length of time with doctor was 'about right'	UK	78		
	USA	74		

Source: Donelan, Blendon et al.[10]

Whereas nearly half of the American patients spent more than 15 minutes with their physician at the time of their last visit, two-thirds of British patients were given less than ten minutes, and 31 per cent 'five minutes or less'. Yet about three-quarters of both American and British patients regarded the length of their visit as 'about right'.

This seemingly cultural phenomenon is further evidence that international comparison of opinions (as distinct from facts) is fraught with problems of interpretation. The National Health Service in the UK has a bedrock of support from people who not only believe in its sanctity but are basically satisfied with the treatment which they and their families have personally received. The biggest obstacle to fundamental reform of the NHS is that the British patient is inclined to accept less in the way of health care than French or German or American patients who want much *more* than they would get in the UK—where the deficiencies in the NHS are made up for by a little grumbling.

It was Lynn Payer who remarked famously in her book, *Medicine and Culture*[11] that '[t]he most striking characteristic of British medicine is its economy. The British do less of nearly everything.'

Such a policy would be totally unacceptable in France. Both the public and the authorities are intensely and introspectively concerned about the state of health of the individual and of society at large. In short, the French demand more and provide more than the British. In its annual household survey in 1998, the health research organisation CREDES reported on a sample of 23,035 persons, representative of 95 per cent of households in metropolitan France. According to their report, during one month, 33 per cent of interviewees had visited a doctor 'at least once': 19 per cent visited a GP, eight per cent a specialist, and six per cent visited both—'at least once'.[12]

One third of the population at the doctor's in one month! With this level of access, professional attention and treatment—most of it reimbursed—it is no surprise that the French population expresses a high degree of satisfaction with its healthcare system. Moreover, as observed in the preceding chapter, French health care also produces superior outcomes.

The Relevance Of Opinion Surveys To Healthcare Rationing

Two aspects are worth exploring: firstly, the public's reaction to actual rationing or to the threat of rationing; and secondly, whether the public favours or objects to discrimination between different groups of patients in order to achieve rationing goals.

Answers to the first question can only be inferred: in most countries, healthcare rationing either does not exist, or it is not recognised as such, or it exists but is denied. From the satisfaction surveys described earlier, it may be reasonable to deduce that France and Germany will basically reject rationing when it comes to the crunch. The American healthcare system is highly flexible and will tolerate grey-area practices up to a point. When that point is passed, Americans will seek changes by means of a blend of political pressure, lawsuits, legislative action, and market forces.

There is published evidence about the second aspect. The French public does not favour prioritisation between groups of patients. In a 1997 survey, 54 per cent of respondents (range 51-58 per cent according to age group) were against 'the state giving priority to certain population groups in its health policy'. Very little support was given to prioritising babies, youth, the elderly or the handicapped. The only significant support (25 per cent) was for 'the most deprived' (les plus démunis').[13]

The British situation is more complex. For years, the existence of rationing was denied; now it is admitted. The level of satisfaction with the NHS has fallen appreciably during the 1990s, yet patients remain on the whole satisfied with the treatment they and their families are receiving.

Throughout the period 1984-1996, the British public considered health to be top priority for 'extra government spending': 45-56 per cent favoured health compared with 20-28 per cent for the next highest priority, education.[14]

A poll on the subject of health rationing by Social & Community Planning Research in 1998 asked respondents to compare a 30-year-old with an equally sick 70-year-old on a waiting list for the same heart operation. Which patient *would* and which patient *should* be operated on first? The question itself is revealing, because such a waiting list would not be the crux of a medical dilemma in France or Germany unless the heart operation were an organ transplant. In the UK, however, the question is a serious one and the answers provide food for thought.

Table 2.3.6
Who **Is** *and Who* **Should** *be Given Priority, UK 1998*
% of responses

Patient's Age	30 years	70 years	Age makes no difference
Who *does* get priority?	51	8	33
Who *should* get priority?	32	7	55

Source: Royal Commission.[15]

A majority of British respondents were of the opinion that ageism exists in the NHS. Only one-third believed that 'age would make no difference'. Opinions on what *should* happen were the reverse: a majority considered that age should make no difference, whereas one-third supported discrimination in favour of the younger patient.

On the other hand, questions specifically enquiring whether respondents favoured cutting down on expensive treatments or services in the NHS and using the savings to provide cheaper care for more people, evoked very negative responses. Fifteen per cent or less favoured cutting down on heart transplants, long-term nursing care of the elderly, or intensive care for premature babies.

The relevance of these poll results is their implication that the act of rationing in the NHS is unpopular with the British public. Expert talk about the 'inevitability' of rationing cuts very little ice. The public recognises that rationing exists and wants less of it. Its strongest belief is that health is top priority and that 'government should spend more on the NHS'. When it comes to how this should be implemented, however, decision makers need to be wary of the 'hypothetical purchase' proposition. What the public says about 'more tax for more health care' and how it votes could be separate and inconsistent choices. On the other hand, after 20 years of recoil from the high tax regimes of the 15 years between 1964 and 1979, a turning point is not inconceivable. Perhaps the day will come when 'more tax for more health care' will be tolerated or even welcomed at the ballot box. So far, however, there is no evidence of a renewed love of taxation. Indeed, the blockade of oil refineries over prices and taxes of September 2000 suggests the reverse.

Oddly, neither the pollsters nor the public seem to be aware of, or willing to accept, the possibility that 'more government spending and more tax' is not the only nor necessarily the best solution. On the subject of health care, public opinion is on a monorail without branch lines. That is the British political dilemma.

4

The United Kingdom: A Rationing Climate

If health managers and economists really believe they appear to society at large as more credible or less absurd than doctors when speaking on its behalf, they have completely lost touch with reality.   *J. Tudor Hart, 1998*

The healthcare climate in the United Kingdom is insular. It lives in a storm zone of its own creation: the National Health Service. Everything revolves around the myth of the NHS. In politics, openly expressed doubts about its absolute and eternal validity will cast a politician into outer darkness. Even the Thatcher government—the most radical in the UK since the Attlee government of 1945-50 which set up the NHS—had to struggle desperately to prove to an incredulous electorate in the 1980s that 'The NHS is safe in our hands'. Belief in a myth will permit the faithful to discount reality.

That is not being flippant. The rationing climate in the UK is tied to the myth of the NHS, its inviolability, and its ultimate sanctity in the eyes of the people and of health experts alike. The myth dictates that rationing is worth enduring if it will help to keep the NHS virginally 'intact'. Of course, everybody knows that the NHS is underfunded and that rationing is therefore *inevitable*. All that is required of the experts is that they should tell us how to ration health care fairly and effectively.

At this point it is worth pausing and asking: how did this myth in a hair shirt come into being?

Pathways To Rationing In The NHS

Six contributory factors may have acted as building blocks over the past half-century. Progressively they may have cemented rationing into the fabric of the NHS and protected it with an aura of untouchability. They are:

i)   Almost total dependence of funding on taxation

ii)   Underfunding

iii) Abnormally low user charges

iv)   Distaste for supplementary forms of health insurance

v)   The 'efficiency delusion'

vi)   A tolerant public with modest expectations

i) *Taxation*

The NHS is funded approximately 80 per cent from general taxation and a further 12 per cent from National Insurance; the balance of about eight per cent is made up of user charges and private health insurance. In its overwhelming reliance on taxation, the UK is not unique in Europe (Scandinavian systems are similar in this respect), but it is very different from France and Germany where health care is funded primarily by social insurance.[1]

Whether taxation as a source of healthcare funding is better or worse than social insurance in principle is not the issue here. Both methods have their pluses and their minuses, their advocates and their opponents. The UK's taxation base has in the last 20 years become a political millstone, an obstacle to funding on an adequate scale, and an encouragement to turn to rationing. If social insurance has proved to be a headache for German and French employers and their international competitiveness, taxation (being less flexible, and unpopular into the bargain) has left successive governments in a cleft stick: they can either raise the tax burden or hold back healthcare spending.

During the first three decades of the NHS, high levels of direct personal taxation were accepted by the British electorate. That changed during the 1980s and 90s when politicians found that their chances of election were slight without a promise to cut direct personal taxes, or at least not to raise them. This has left the NHS in a financially precarious situation, dependent on the rate of growth of taxable incomes and on the degree of priority given to health in government expenditure.

The result has been drift towards rationing. Governments have doled out extra funds to the NHS like aspirins, as a form of crisis-calming relief. These gestures have had little practical impact on the basic problem. Even the massive increases announced in March 2000 do not change the underlying principle: tax funding means underfunding in the long run unless rapid and uninterrupted economic growth is achieved or voters can be persuaded to pay more tax.

ii) *Underfunding*

The NHS is chronically underfunded and has been so from the start.

> The estimates of likely expenditure on the NHS, made by the founding fathers, were too low and the Treasury had to find additional resources as early as 1948 to fill the gap. The imposition of an expenditure ceiling followed quickly, as did controls over manpower.[2]

Under-estimating current and future demand for health care was a serious error from the outset. The belief that the NHS would, by improving the people's health, depress the quantity of care required to meet a gradually falling level of demand was foolish even at the time. Yet in a society that rejected the inequalities of pre-war medicine and was accustomed to war-time rationing, it seemed fitting to expect that the public would be grateful for a modestly funded NHS. And so it proved. The public was exceedingly grateful, so much so that it made prolific use of the NHS and took it to its heart where it has remained ever since—underfunded.

Evidently, persistent underfunding is a precursor of rationing and promotes a climate of opinion that regards rationing as a valid and necessary means of balancing the books. In the UK, rationing has also aggravated the *need* for rationing by inducing shortages of family doctors, specialists, nurses and other skilled health professionals.

iii) *Abnormally low user charges*

User charges—or co-payment by patients at the point of use—have been discussed in Part I-2(vi) as a method of cost containment. They have been kept relatively low in most countries, partly because they are unpopular and partly because they can deter patients from seeking necessary medical advice and treatment. In the UK, they are *abnormally* low.

Mossialos and Le Grand[3] have estimated that user charges make a 3.2 per cent contribution to healthcare finance in the UK, 7.3 per cent in Germany, 16.5 per cent (including voluntary health insurance) in France, in a range of 17-21 per cent in Scandinavia, and 31 per cent in Italy. Compared with France and Germany, British user charges are as follows:

Table 2.4.1
User Charges 1996-2000

Service	UK	France	Germany
GP visit	nil	30%	nil
Specialist	nil	30% (25% at public hospital)	nil
Hospital in-patient	nil	20% (+ 'hotel' charge)	DM 17 ($10) per day for first 14 days (DM 14 in former East Germany)
Drug Prescription	£6.00 ($9.50) per item prescribed	0-35-65% depending on drug	DM 8-9-10 ($4.50-5.70) depending on pack size

Source: Mossialos and Le Grand.[4]
Note: Pharmaceuticals and German charges updated by author

In the UK, user charges are negligible. Even the prescription charge is not what it appears to be, because 83 per cent of prescriptions are exempt. There are no NHS user charges for ambulatory or institutional care.

In Germany, user charges were substantially raised in 1997, but the prescription charge was subsequently reduced by DM 1. Exemptions are less prolific than in the UK.

France has heavy charges which patients must actually pay, but most can be recovered by the 85 per cent of the population that has taken out supplementary health insurance with a *mutuelle* or similar insurer. The true user charge for most of the population is therefore the supplementary insurance premium.

It could be argued that the absence of effective user charges in the UK is a form of generosity and the very opposite of rationing. Such a view is too simplistic. User charges can make a useful if limited contribution to the funding of health care. To deprive the system of that contribution is to intensify the pressure to ration. It is also an abdication of political courage not even to attempt to persuade the electorate that moderate user charges are a necessary component of a modern health service.

iv) *Distaste for supplementary forms of health insurance*

The French system of *assurance complémentaire* has been criticised for encouraging profligate consumption. In fact it relieves the state of a considerable financial burden by introducing a buffer between national health insurance and users. It is the British system which encourages irresponsible consumption by charging the user nothing and rejecting the supplementary insurance option. If actual consumption is high in France and low in the UK, that is attributable mainly to differences in national medical culture rather than to the supplementary insurance mechanism (see Part II-5).

In the UK, supplementary insurance exists in the private sector, but operates above all by enabling patients to avoid waiting lists for elective surgery and to choose more expensive 'hotel' options as in-patients. In other words, it provides an escape route from rationing in the NHS for those who can afford the premiums. This form of supplementary insurance receives no encouragement from government policy in the UK.

v) *The 'efficiency delusion'*

In official circles, the argument runs that the NHS is not really under-funded, and that rationing could be avoided by strenuous efforts to improve the efficiency of the service.

That is a delusion. It is on a par with the assertion that you can shake off your clinical depression if you will just 'pull yourself together'. Of course, the efficiency of the service—of any service—can always be improved. No one would deny that. The delusion springs from three separate beliefs:

i)   that the scope for greater efficiency is *vast*

ii)   that results of great magnitude can be achieved *quickly*

iii) that such efficiency gains will solve the underfunding crisis of the NHS and make rationing unnecessary

The first two beliefs are typical of inward-looking attitudes towards the NHS. International comparisons tend, on the contrary, to demonstrate that, at least in terms of productivity, the NHS is a relatively efficient organisation. It also produces reasonably good results with its very limited resources.

Table 2.4.2
Service Ratios, mid-1990s

Ratio	UK	France	Germany
Practising doctors/100,000 population	156	285	328
Registered nurses/100,000 population	450	590	950
Hospitals, average length of stay, days	9.8	11.2	14.3
Hospitals, length of stay in acute beds, days	4.8	5.9	12.1
Hospitals, beds per 100,000 population	4.9	8.7	7.3
Hospitals, acute care beds per 100,000 popul.	2.0	4.6	6.3
Annual expenditure *per capita*, in $PPP			
Hospitals	521	902	796
Physicians	184	237	375
Pharmaceuticals	218	337	289

Sources: *OECD Health Data 99* and other OECD-related sources.

On each of these ratios, UK input of resources is far below that of France and Germany. If anything, the NHS deserves applause for the results that it has been able to achieve with inadequate inputs.

Efficiency in health care is a double-edged sword. Striving for greater productivity is both welcome and ultimately necessary for the survival of the system and the patient. Yet there comes a point where an obsessive quest for efficiency will damage the quality of health care. The best efficiency ratios cannot automatically be equated with the most effective medicine.

The political uproar about managed care in the USA (see Part II-7) is precisely over this conflict between efficiency and quality. What managed care organisations are best at is financial efficiency. At first, this produced useful savings, because health care under fee-for-service conditions had been rather inefficient. By 1998, the quality of managed care was being seriously questioned. In their survey of public discontent, Donelan, Blendon *et al*,[5] reported that 28 per cent of US respondents under traditional insurance declared that 'medical care received over the past six months was excellent', compared with only 16 per cent under managed care. 'Difficulties in seeing specialists and consultants' were cited by 25 per cent of the traditionally insured and by 40 per cent of those in managed care. These are the ragged edges of efficiency.

The 'efficiency delusion' can only aggravate the tendency to cut corners on the quality front and to reinforce the rationing impulse that springs from inadequate resources. There is, however, a difference between eliminating inefficiency and maximising efficiency. The NHS can benefit from the former but may already have gone too far in the direction of the latter, to the point where maximisation is achieved by cutting back resources. The result is not efficiency but rationing.

vi) *A tolerant public with modest expectations*

Surveys of public satisfaction have been described in Part II-3. They show that the British public in 1996 was somewhat less satisfied and much more dissatisfied with 'the way health care is run' than the public in France and Germany. On the other hand, between half and two-thirds of UK patients considered in 1998 that the care which they and their families have recently received was 'excellent' or 'very good'. These contradictory findings might be explained by the 'grumble hypothesis' set out in Part II-3: we complain about what 'they up there seem to be doing but, mind you, our Dr Smith is a gem of a GP!'

The tolerance of the British public is legendary. Their expectations may be rising but they remain relatively modest. The rationing climate in the NHS is held up in France and Germany as a warning of what must not be allowed to happen there. As an example, in July1999, during a debate on health reform in the German *Bundestag*, a health expert from the opposition FDP predicted that Germany would have:

...Rationierung, Wartelisten und Altersgrenzen für bestimmte medizinische Leistungen, wie es sie in Grossbritannien gebe. Er forderte stattdessen, die Eigenverantwortung der Versicherten zu stärken.

...rationing, waiting lists and age limits for certain medical services as in Great Britain. He demanded instead that measures be taken to strengthen the responsibility of the insured.[6]

The British public may no longer believe that 'the NHS is the best health service in the world', but the idealistic aura surrounding its birth in 1948 has not faded.

Admirable! Yet the public's strong attachment to the NHS as an 'ideal' system has made it politically hazardous for any government to tinker with the fundamental principles of the service, let alone reform it or update it radically. The public dislikes rationing, but is evidently willing to tolerate it, if toleration will help to 'save' the NHS. Paradoxically, the public's nostalgia for the idealism of the founders' era reinforces a rationing climate whose manifestations in the real world are unpopular. Politically, it is a vicious circle.

The Symptoms Of Rationing

The general shortage of physical resources in the NHS has already been described. Three specific symptoms are explored below:

i)   Waiting lists
ii)   Outbreaks of anecdotal fury in the media
iii)   Resistance to medical and pharmaceutical innovation, leading to 'postcode rationing'

These symptoms are cited because they distinguish the UK sharply from France, Germany and—except perhaps for (ii)—the USA. Waiting lists in the NHS are long and persistent. There is a continuous flow of media noise about deficiencies in health care on the NHS, spiced with sensational 'human interest' content. The flu epidemic 'that never was' of January 2000 is a representative example of anecdotal fury. As for the third symptom, the NHS is notorious for what Nick Bosanquet has sardonically described in psychiatric terms as its innovation phobia:

> The NHS may be beginning to suffer from a problem that might be called 'innovation phobia'. Any new innovation is regarded with great suspicion because it might raise costs or attract more patients. The NHS now provides a paradox of a health service where many live in fear that new ways will be found of curing disease.[7]

In its multiple ramifications, this innovation phobia is also one of the pathways to postcode rationing.

i) Waiting lists and waiting times

Waiting lists are not widely investigated or reported in France and Germany because, exceptional circumstances apart, they are not regarded as a serious problem. Waiting for an organ graft is an exception throughout the industrialised world, as described in Part I-4.

Donelan, Blendon et al,[8] in their survey of the public, compared 'waiting times for non-emergency surgery for themselves or a family member' in the US and UK. They reported as follows:

Table 2.4.3
Waiting Times for Non-Emergency Surgery, 1998

Waiting time	% of respondents	
	UK	USA
None/less than a month	30	70
1 - 3.9 months	36	28
4 months or longer	33	1

Source: Donelan, Blendon *et al.*[9]

One-third of a 'nationally representative' sample of 'non-institutional-ised' British respondents reported having to wait four months or longer, compared with one per cent of Americans. Waiting for non-emergency surgery is a British disease and directly attributable to rationing in the NHS. Inadequate financial input has created a chronic shortage of physical and professional resources in relation to demand.

NHS waiting times are a striking example of a 'Double Whammy': patients have to be referred to specialists by their GPs and wait for an appointment. When the specialist endorses surgical intervention, there is then a further waiting time before hospital admission as an in-patient.

At 31 March 1999, there was a waiting list for elective surgery at NHS hospitals in England of 1,070,000 patients. Of these, 270,000 had been waiting for admission for more than six months.[10]

That is rationing in action.

In 1997/98, on average 19 per cent of NHS patients had to wait longer than three months after referral before obtaining a first appointment with a specialist. Thereafter, 29 per cent of patients had not been admitted as in-patients within three months of the decision to admit.

That is rationing in action.

The best access to specialists was recorded for paediatricians and mental illness (six per cent waiting more than three months); the worst for trauma/orthopaedics (36 per cent) and plastic surgery (31 per cent). For in-patient admission, the best access was achieved in paediatrics (four per cent waiting more than three months) and gastroenterology (ten per cent); the worst for trauma/orthopaedics (54 per cent) and ophthalmology (52 per cent).[11]

ii) *Rationing and the media*

The misfortunes of NHS patients have always attracted media attention, because bad news makes good copy. In late-1999 and early-2000, interest in bad health service news became feverish. Hardly a day would pass without articles with human interest stories that would make readers shudder. Here are four mild examples from the quality press (*fictitious names substituted*):

Heart man on one-year waiting list given six months to live.[12]

Last Monday, Peter Ford was out of bed by 5.30am, anxiously preparing for the treatment he hoped would finally cure his cancerous tumour. Ford, 41, married with three young children ... [Despite his appointment, he had to wait three more days before a bed could be found and treatment could begin.][13]

My father has had his operation cancelled. He needs a hip replacement and has endured considerable pain and disability for well over a year. He has been told he will have a permanent limp which will inevitably cause his other hip to deteriorate.[14]

James Williams, 33, went to hospital complaining of symptoms of chest pains, raging temperature and a headache. He was sent home and told to wrap up warm with plenty of hot drinks. But he collapsed and died just hours later. 'I know they are snowed under with people suffering from flu but he was sent home to die', his mother Joan said.[15]

That is rationing in action.

It was the outbreak of influenza which peaked in late-December 1999 and early-January 2000 that pushed media interest in the misery of NHS patients to an appalling climax. The NHS was heavily outgunned by the flu bug. There were not enough available hospital beds, and intensive care units were stretched beyond breaking point: only two such beds were available in NHS hospitals in the whole of London on 28 December 1999 (*Financial Times*, 29 December 1999). Patients with other serious conditions were crowded out by influenza victims. Some were dumped on trolleys in hospital corridors; others were shunted around the regions. The beds were there, but not the registered nurses needed to look after patients. Field days for the media ...

That is rationing in action.

The government's response was inept. Spin doctors quickly invented the alibi of a flu *epidemic*, so serious that it would throw *any* health-care system off-course. In fact, the flu crisis never reached levels that met the official medical definition of an *epidemic* outbreak, but it made good soundbites for a few days. The media then began a concentrated attack on British health care: the lamentable state of the NHS, the government's broken promises, the funding system, the rationing mindset, the excuses, even the treasured myth of the NHS itself.

The government responded with somewhat improvised emergency announcements. The Prime Minister promised to raise health expenditure as a percentage of GDP to the European average within five years. When this was interpreted as a pledge, government spokespersons hurriedly converted it into an 'aspiration'. It was panic stations in the ivory tower of healthcare rationing.

Practical action followed when the Chancellor presented his national budget to Parliament in March 2000. This contained a massive cash injection into the NHS (£2 billion for 2000-2001) and *real* increases of six per cent annually for the following four years.[16] The aim to raise healthcare spending to the European average remains an 'aspiration' with major arithmetical disputes among experts about the precise financial input required to achieve it.

The budget was followed in July 2000 by the government's NHS Plan which is briefly discussed within the rationing context of this study in Part III, Chapter 2.

iii) Rationing and resistance to innovation

> There is legitimate concern that preoccupation with cost will distract from the value of innovative new medicines, and that this will indirectly discourage therapeutic research.[17]

The UK has an excellent record of innovative achievement in surgery, medical devices and pharmaceuticals. The NHS, on the other hand, has a weak and deteriorating record of accepting (let alone welcoming) innovation. Its innovation phobia is not sporadic but endemic; it is not accidental but intentional; it is not haphazard but organised. It has been progressively built into the control procedures of the healthcare system: it is rationing in action.

The case of innovative pharmaceuticals is illustrative. Once again, it is necessary to distinguish between normal cost containment and rationing. Every healthcare system practises cost containment of drug expenditure and most will trespass into the grey area between expenditure restraint and rationing (see Part I-3). The NHS crossed the additional bridge into rationing some years ago.

Horizon scanning

One of the first clear symptoms was the setting up of so-called horizon scanning. This eminently sensible management tool is used in the NHS to scan the horizon for new drugs roughly five years before such drugs are expected to reach the market. Horizon scanners follow them through their development phases in order to assess their potential impact on NHS expenditure. Nothing wrong with that. It is a sign of good management to maintain consistent awareness of trends in innovation and their financial implications.

The problem is not the procedure of horizon scanning but the policy and attitude of those for whom the horizon is being scanned. For them, the practice acts as a financial hurricane warning and a red alert for action stations on rationing. The motive behind horizon scanning is not to prompt the system to procure the resources needed to pay for innovative drugs, because that would not be practicable in a cash-strapped, underfunded NHS. Instead, it is to warn the controllers to get ready to unsheathe their pruning knives.

In the NHS, innovative drugs are not regarded as medically beneficial but as a budget-busting menace. They were actually described as a *'threat'* by the authors of a description of drug budget management in Glasgow:

> Twin threats come from the introduction of new expensive medicines for previously untreatable conditions, and from the increasing, high volume use of drugs with important public health applications, for example angiotensin-converting enzyme inhibiting drugs,* lipid lowering agents, and antipsychotic drugs.[18]

The target of 'threat' management happens to be a trio of major pharmaceutical innovations representing proven advances in drug therapy. Large-scale outcome trials have shown that ACE-inhibitors and statins (lipid, i.e. cholesterol-lowering drugs) significantly reduce mortality from various forms of heart disease, while the new antipsychotic drugs mark an important advance in the treatment of schizophrenia. The Glasgow authors fully recognise this, but as budget controllers they are caught in the meshes of NHS rationing. It is a curious form of healthcare prioritisation.

National Institute for Clinical Excellence (NICE)

> NICE is the British Government's mechanism for rationing the availability of new medical technology in the NHS.[19]

Most of the reforms of the NHS which took effect on 1 March 1999 are not specifically concerned with rationing, but the setting up of the National Institute for Clinical Excellence is relevant to the issue.

The purpose of NICE is exquisitely ambivalent. Officially NICE will indeed promote the cause of clinical excellence. To do so, it has a mandate to assess all new and existing medicines and other clinical interventions in the NHS and make recommendations which physicians will be expected to heed. Why this form of assessment should be necessary for *new* drugs whose safety and efficacy have already been approved as a condition of registration by the British Medicines Control Agency or the European Medicines Evaluation Agency, has not been made explicit.

However, the government's White Paper which projected the setting up of NICE hinted at an economic function whilst making it clear that NICE would not be controlling prices. In somewhat turgid prose, the White Paper warned that:

---

*   ACE inhibitors.

... where evidence of [cost-effectiveness] has not become available at the point
that a product comes to market, NICE may recommend that in the first instance
the NHS channels its use through well controlled research studies.[20]

The *precise* meaning of this thinly veiled threat is nicely obscure, but
the general drift is clear enough: pharmacoeconomic studies, although
not mandatory, had best be provided as evidence of cost-effectiveness,
or else ...*delay*. If and when the studies are submitted, their validity
can then be the subject of prolonged disputes, causing further ...*delay*.
NICE may then demand additional studies to clarify areas of uncertainty and involving yet more ...*delay*. NICE's resources in the face of
the prospective volume and scale of its tasks are also uncertain and
may necessitate yet further ...*delay*.

To delay the entry of new products into healthcare markets is a
classical grey-area tool of cost containment. Often, it is hard to tell
whether the grounds for delay have substance or are dragged in. When
this deprives patients of innovative medicines for significant periods
of time, it can reasonably be interpreted as a symptom of rationing.
The delay cannot be justified on medical grounds, because these were
fully assessed prior to registration. The sticking point is cost and its
impact on the NHS budget. Delay nicely postpones that 'threat'.

The management of NICE has consistently emphasised its support
for innovation where it contributes cost-effectively to clinical excellence, and there is no reason to doubt its commitment.

Nevertheless, judging by the Institute's appraisals and recommendations during its first year, NICE is evidently fulfilling a grey-area role
by causing delay and uncertainty among prescribers, patients
organisations and the research-based pharmaceutical industry. It
would be premature to describe NICE as an instrument of outright
rationing. Some of its recommendations to date will actually increase
costs in the NHS, for example in the use of taxanes for ovarian and
breast cancer. However, positive guidance from NICE for the latter
emerged only after the Appeals Panel upheld appeals against its
original recommendation by the pharmaceutical company Bristol
Myers Squibb and a cancer charity.[21]

A more controversial test of NICE's role and policy judgment (as yet
unresolved at the time of writing) arose from the Institute's prelimi-
nary recommendation in June 2000 against the use in the NHS of
beta-interferon for the treatment of multiple sclerosis (MS) except for
patients who are already on the drug. The negative appraisal was
based on NICE's view that the medical benefit of beta-interferon was
insufficient to justify its high cost. By the end of August, seven appeals
against NICE's final recommendation had been lodged. The MS
Society, working on behalf of patients, was also reported to be
considering further action *via* human rights legislation, because 'only

two-three per cent of [MS] patients received beta-interferon in the UK compared with 10-12 per cent of MS patients in countries such as the US, Germany and France'.[22]

Whatever the outcome, the beta-interferon case exposes a disturbing conflict between medical ethics, patients' rights, the demand for cost-effectiveness, and rationing in the NHS. Physicians, patients and pharmaceutical companies want beta-interferon to be available for those patients who can derive benefit from it. NICE interposes a cost-effectiveness hurdle of questionable validity for a disease as serious and difficult to treat as MS.

> Edith Newell told Tony Blair this year that she was 'devastated' to have been refused beta-interferon because of the cost. The Prime Minister, taking part in a televised debate in the hospital where Mrs Newell is treated for multiple sclerosis, assured her that the appraisal by the National Institute for Clinical Excellence would solve the problem.

> Yesterday's news that the drug will probably be banned on the NHS has appalled Mrs Newell. 'We are devastated', she said. 'It rules out hope for those with MS who are not already on it.'[23]

Quite apart from misery caused to therapeutically eligible patients, it is medically nonsensical to allow the drug to continue to be used for existing NHS patients whilst withholding it from new patients. That can be explained only as a *political* decision: can we avoid an otherwise unavoidable furore if we refrain from actually taking patients off this drug in the face of individual doctors' judgment of benefit to individual patients?

The political content of NICE's recommendation takes it straight into rationing territory. Of the four rationing criteria, two are clearly at work: denial of quality treatment and blatant discrimination between patients regardless of need. A final decision, too, can be based on political considerations rather than cost-effectiveness, because the Secretary of State for Health retains the power to reject the judgment of NICE if he considers it to be politically expedient to do so.

It seems reasonable to conclude that NICE's record to date shows it to be an instrument of delay, poised on the threshold of rationing. The recommendations follow the Institute's terms of reference. Officials are doing their duty. It is the concept of NICE that is at fault. The Institute is misconceived as a judge of innovation. Ambivalently interposed between the NHS and its doctors, NICE sets out to declare 'clinical excellence' whilst operating an 'affordability' screen that rations without appearing to do so.

Postcode Rationing

A more overt form of rationing is by postcode. Health authorities in different parts of the country may individually decide that *their* budget cannot afford the cost of a particular treatment, or can afford it only for a limited number of patients. Were the patient resident in an area served by a more generous health authority, that patient might be receiving that treatment under the NHS. Again, beta-interferon features prominently in this controversial practice:

Couple will sell house to buy drug for MS son.
... Health Authority has told the family that it cannot afford the annual £ 10,000 ($ 16,000) bill for the drug. It funds Beta Interferon for 11 of the 63 patients assessed for the treatment in its area.
NB: The couple's son 'has been passed suitable for the drug'.[24]

This is rationing in its most disturbing form, with an arbitrary cut-off point at the eleventh patient out of 63, leaving an undisclosed number of 'suitable' patients without innovative drug therapy in a rich country. Beta-interferon is the first approved drug treatment specifically for multiple sclerosis. In 1999, it was described as 'difficult or near impossible to obtain in south-west England, Buckinghamshire, Nottinghamshire, northern England and most ...of Scotland'.[25]

There is widespread condemnation of postcode rationing, and the government wants NICE to put a stop to it. It is difficult to see how NICE could intervene to prohibit the practice, because the institute is not responsible for financial allocations, budget management or drug pricing. Numerous commentators have pointed out that postcode rationing will continue unless NICE's guidance, when positive, is backed by additional NHS funds. That may well happen for treatments involving modest additional funds. Will it also occur for expensive, high-volume treatments?

In other words, rationing will come full circle unless its causes are removed. Is it not time to face the fact that postcode rationing is an aberration that springs directly from chronic underfunding of the National Health Service? Prescribing guidelines with a *medical* basis for patient selection are a reasonable method of avoiding wasteful, inappropriate and ineffective use of costly drugs. The postcode route, with or without NICE, is the unintended consequence of a health service that sees rationing, *not* the reform of funding, as the answer to its plight.

5

France: Crisis in Plenty

L'État-providence actuel est en retard d'adaptation. Non pas par rapport aux risques de demain, mais par rapport à ceux d'aujourd' hui... L'État-providence est en crise parce qu'il ne correspond plus à l'univers actuel des risques.

The present-day welfare state is slow to adapt, not to tomorrow's risks but to those of today... The welfare state is in crisis because it no longer reflects the real world of risks.

Denis Kessler[1]

Crisis in the welfare state is not confined to France. Its repercussions in the UK have been described in the preceding chapter. Those in Germany and in public sector health care in the USA follow in the next two. Yet, as French public sector health care lurches from one financial crisis to the next, there appears to be little or no rationing in France. This paradox is worth exploring.

Health Care In Abundance

A fundamental difference between French and British health care is that the crisis in France is one of super-abundance whereas that in the UK is caused by chronic shortages. Another difference between the two countries is that French experts are almost unanimous in criticising their healthcare system, whereas British experts treat the NHS reverently and with benign indulgence.

The French authorities are desperately trying to contain health expenditure by every conceivable method of financial control. The British authorities, equally desperate, are driven to ration the provision of care. Although French control measures are increasingly straying into the grey area between cost containment and rationing, the rationing climate of the UK would be unacceptable in France. Conversely, the elaborate stranglehold of official controls on which France relies, is alien to the British way of dealing more pragmatically with critical situations.

An excessive supply of healthcare resources in France is of long standing. It is centred on a surplus of physicians and hospital facilities. Between 1975 and 1997, the number of practising physicians in France nearly tripled, although the rate of increase slowed in the 1990s, and numbers fell for the first time in 1997.[2]

73

The adoption in 1971 of a *numerus clausus* for medical students drastically reduced their number from 8,588 in 1972 to 3,750 in 1995.[3] The surplus of doctors is gradually coming under control. For the present, however, it continues to stimulate consumption in a system that is based almost entirely on fee-for-service remuneration. Moreover, French patients are free to choose their GPs as well as their specialists to whom they have direct access. They will tend to gravitate towards doctors who prescribe liberally. '*L'attachement des Français à la liberté du choix limite les possibilités d'autres solutions*' ('The attachment of the French to freedom of choice limits the scope for other solutions').[4]

The density of physicians in France is unevenly spread. By and large, it is highest in the south and in urban areas, and lowest in the north and in rural areas. In 1997, there were four rural *départements* in which no new GP practice had been opened during the year. Against an average density of 164 GPs per 100,000 population, the range is from 113 in Eure to 291 in Paris. Even more crassly, the spread of specialists (average density 155) is between 64 in Haute-Loire and 509 in Paris.[5]

Thus, although there is over-supply of physicians nationally, there are pockets of inadequate provision locally. The same applies to some segments of the specialist establishment which, overall, is heavily in surplus. By 1997, 48.8 per cent of all practising physicians were specialists, compared with 39 per cent in 1985.[6] Yet there are not enough anaesthetists:

> *Annulation de la lithotritie deux jours par semaine pendant six semaines, fermeture d'une salle d'opération sur quatre au Pavillon V, des consultations d'anaesthésie supprimées, des délais d'intervention chirurgicale atteignant trois semaines ... parce que le médecin anaesthésiste qui les assure remplace ses confrères dans les blocs opératoires.*

> Cancellation of lithotripter sessions twice a week for six weeks, closure of one in four operating theatres in Pavilion V, no anaesthesia consultations, postponement of surgical interventions by three weeks ... because the anaesthetist physician responsible for these is standing in for his colleagues in the operating areas.[7]

One might as well be in England. However, anaesthesia is one of the few areas of medicine and surgery where there is an acknowledged shortage of specialists in France. Overall, the hospital sector is grossly in surplus:

> France is grappling with serious problems of over-capacity at state-owned hospitals, which account for 65 per cent of total hospital bed capacity.[8]

The number of hospital beds has been cut back by six per cent during the first half of the 1990s, but hospital closures in order to rationalise the system are extremely difficult to bring off in practice:

Les fermetures d'hôpitaux ou de services hospitaliers se heurtent cependant à des oppositions politiques locales, compte tenu à la fois de la sensibilité de la population aux conditions de l'accès aux soins et du rôle des hôpitaux sur l'emploi et l'ensemble de l'économie locale.

Closure of hospitals and hospital services, however, runs into local political opposition in view of popular sensitivity to the conditions of access to care and the part played by hospitals in employment and in the local economy overall.[9]

Cost containment in France: *'J'enrage ...'*

The French healthcare system is generous to a fault, but it is not economically efficient. That is why patients love it and why the authorities are perpetually trying to refine their mechanisms of cost containment and control.

National health insurance (*Assurance-Maladie*) continues to defy the efforts of successive governments to end its annual deficits so as to bring social security finance as a whole into balance or surplus. Although the health insurance deficit was halved between 1996 and 1998 and the *Ministère de l'Emploi et de la Solidarité* has forecast near-balance in 2000,[10] prospects will remain precarious as demand tends to rise, in the long run, above officially planned targets and limits.

The most important form of cost control is the *Objectif National des Dépenses d'Assurance-Maladie* (ONDAM) or national target for health insurance expenditure. On first hearing the expression ONDAM, Professor Jean-Pierre Bader confessed that he thought it sounded like a Flemish curse or a god of the Vikings.[11] He soon discovered that it is the 'envelope' of total healthcare expenditure which, in accordance with an annually renewed law of social security finance (*Loi de Financement pour la Sécurité Sociale*) must not grow by more than a specified percentage. The target is sub-divided into separate 'envelopes' for hospitals, ambulatory care, pharmaceuticals and numerous other healthcare goods and services. For the year 2000, the ONDAM for national health insurance was fixed at 2.5 per cent above actual expenditure in 1999. Each sector is required to respect the ONDAM, with threats of penalty payments for exceeding the target.

J'enrage littéralement quand j'entends un décideur affirmer qu'il n'y a pas lieu d'augmenter les dépenses de santé.

I literally fly into a temper when I hear a decision maker's assertion that it is inappropriate to raise health expenditure.[12]

If only British academics would occasionally fly into a Gallic temper instead of preaching the virtues of rationing...

Professor Bader goes straight to the heart of the matter. What was kidney failure like before dialysis and grafts, he asks, or heart disease before bypass surgery and valve replacement, or arthritis before hip replacement, or 'the fate of the depressed who used to be locked up and can today live with their families'?

When it comes to the crunch, France will pay for major innovation, though not without agonising resistance by the authorities and a surfeit of controls. Innovative pharmaceuticals are a case in point.

Innovative Pharmaceuticals: A Grey Area

Cost containment of prescription drugs perhaps comes nearest to the point where France crosses the borderline into rationing. The control system has certainly strayed deep into the grey area.

Apart from having to abide by the ONDAM, the pharmaceutical industry in France is bound by the *Accord Sectoriel 1999-2002* (Pharmaceutical Sector Agreement) and by complex procedures preceding approval of reimbursement. These involve drug evaluation by the *Commission de la Transparence* and price regulation by the *Comité Economique des Produits de Santé* (Economic Committee) before reimbursement under national health insurance is either granted or refused.

The *Accord Sectoriel* was signed in July 1999 by the Economic Committee and SNIP (*Syndicat National de l'Industrie Pharmaceutique*) on behalf of the industry. It makes some concessions to industrial interests but is basically an instrument of cost containment. It ties reimbursement of drugs directly to the ONDAM and lays down that the Economic Committee will each year unilaterally decide sales growth targets for different classes of reimbursable drugs.

Companies can either negotiate and sign a 'convention' agreement with the Economic Committee or have their drug prices fixed (and probably reduced) by public decree. If sales exceed the target, companies will remit penalty payments covering at least 25 per cent of the excess. These penalties are euphemistically termed 'quantity discounts for everybody'.[13]

In a review of the new medicines policy in France, Professor Claude Le Pen has described the system as 'over-regulated'. Control is now exercised at five separate levels: by total pharmaceutical expenditure, by therapeutic class, by company, by price/volume control of individual products, and by special measures to deal with drugs of low therapeutic value or very fast growth.[14]

When control is carried to these extremes, it almost negates the existence of a pharmaceutical market. Companies will be *punished* for selling too much. The authorities decide at what rate each reimbursable class of prescription drugs is to grow. The *Accord Sectoriel* actually has an appendix that lists the permitted rates of growth by therapeutic class and sub-class in relation to the ONDAM. Each case is reasoned with impeccable logic, but the sum-total creates a make-believe world in which top-down planners pre-emptively fix the advance of medicine and markets in minute detail.

King Canute stood on the seashore and ordered the tide to retreat. We all know what happened to him.

Are Pharmaceuticals Being Rationed In France?

Surprisingly perhaps, one is driven to the conclusion that they are not being rationed. The four essential components of rationing are all missing: there is no shortage of supply; there are no waiting lists and no postcode rationing decisions; there is no denial of quality treatment, and there is no discrimination between patients in the *Accord Sectoriel*. On the other hand, denial of quality can come close to being enforced by other control measures, such as the refusal by the Economic Committee to grant reimbursement at an industrially acceptable price.

In point of fact, the *Accord Sectoriel* reveals a slight but inadequate bias in favour of innovation and quality treatment by allowing rates of growth in excess of the ONDAM for drug classes in which innovation is causing a rapid growth in demand. By contrast, drug categories in which there is 'abusive over-consumption' are to be severely repressed, as are drugs of little or no medical value.

This is further reinforced by a new system for the assessment of the medical value of drugs by the *Commission de la Transparence*. In the past, the Commission was responsible for evaluating new drugs in terms of their contribution to the improvement of therapy (*Amélioration du Service Médical Rendu*: ASMR). To this has now been added an absolute value assessment (*Service Médical Rendu*: SMR). This is to be applied to both old and new drugs. Three levels of SMR are identified: major/important, moderate, and low value; a drug may also be classed as of 'no attributed value'.

This evaluation is medical, not economic, but it will influence the Economic Committee in its decisions on pricing and reimbursement. 'The decree permits a re-evaluation of all products in the same therapeutic class with a view to harmonising their reimbursement status'.[15] 'Harmonising' sounds gentle and sensible, but the actual purpose of the new requirements is to differentiate between products in the same therapeutic class, and to de-list those that are deemed to provide insufficient medical value. A substantial push to exclude many older drugs from reimbursement is expected.

These measures broaden the range and deepen the scope of pharmaceutical cost containment in France. They are designed to limit the state's responsibility for drug reimbursement to a fixed sum related to the ONDAM. Any excess will be paid for, not by patients but by the pharmaceutical industry. Patients will be affected indirectly if reimbursement for new and innovative drugs is refused or delayed on price grounds, or if drug companies opt not to apply for reimbursement. For example, of 60 new drugs which were approved under the European Union's centralised procedure in 1998 and 1999, only 28 were being reimbursed in France on 21 December 1999.[16]

In this sense, the measures are evidently in the grey area between normal cost containment and rationing. They are also widely regarded as sealing the fate of much of what remains of the French-owned pharmaceutical industry, because industrial policy is being harshly subordinated to the priorities of cost containment in health care.

Lessons Of The Past

Successive French governments have fought a losing battle with rising health expenditure over the past 25 years, interspersed with brief victorious interludes. Between 1975 and 1995, a dozen ministers have sought immortality by giving their names to a healthcare 'Plan', from the *Plan Durafour* (1975) which removed the income ceiling for health insurance contribution for the higher paid, to the *Plan Juppé* (1995) which was designed to eliminate health insurance deficits. It led to strikes by health professionals and social unrest, but remained sufficiently intact for the imposition of the ONDAM in the late-1990s.

Numerous explanations have been sought for the endemic state of financial crisis in French national health insurance. Ultimately the most cogent is the popularity of the French system of health care with the electorate. This has forced the authorities to be responsive—up to a point—to demand rather than to ration supply.

> *Au cours des vingt dernières années, l'augmentation des ressources a été la méthode de prédilection des gouvernements pour limiter les déficits de l'Assurance-maladie à court terme. Moins dangereuse que la baisse des prestations...*

> During the last 20 years, governments' preferred method of limiting health insurance deficits in the short term has been *to increase resources*. Politically less dangerous than reducing benefits...[17]

'Politically less dangerous than reducing benefits': that is the crux. In the UK, it is politically less dangerous to ration benefits than to raise taxes. In France, social insurance contributions have been raised steeply from 1.5 per cent of employees' wages and salaries and 2.5 per cent employers' contribution in 1975 to 6.8 per cent and 12.8 per cent, respectively, in 1995. The public has accepted these increases as the price of generous healthcare provision.

By now, this vein may have been exhausted as far as employers are concerned. Not only is their level of contribution regarded as internationally uncompetitive for business and industry, but MEDEF (the employers' federation) has signalled its intention to withdraw from the post-war consensus (*paritarisme*) whereby employers and the trades unions jointly supervised social security finance.[18] Whether this will actually happen or is an opening move in a bargaining round, is uncertain at the time of writing this review. Were it, or anything approaching it, to occur, it could be the start of radical changes in the French social security (including health care) consensus.

By contrast, increases in user charges have been consistently unpopular in France. An early attempt to raise user charges in 1965 had to be reversed after the 'students' revolution' of 1968.Twenty-five years were to elapse before a further serious attempt was made in 1993.[19] Even a moderate move to abolish certain exemptions from the *'ticket modérateur'* (user charge) under the *Plan Séguin* in 1986 was reversed in 1989 by the *Plan Evin*. At the time, the *Plan Séguin* was even blamed as a contributory cause of the ruling party's defeat at the subsequent election. In France, it is politically dangerous to make voters pay for their health care at the point of use—unless they can recover such payments.

The Role Of Supplementary Health Insurance

The need for supplementary insurance (*assurance complémentaire*) in France is primarily the result of the *impasse* reached by the public sector in its perpetual state of financial crisis:

- Patients are basically happy with the French healthcare system

- Their demand for health care is rising and will continue to do so

- Control and efficiency measures in the public sector have consistently failed to achieve more than short-term savings

- The deficit of *Assurance-Maladie* is a drag on the policy of balancing the books of social security as a whole

- Employers are no longer willing to accept further increases in social charges

- Higher out-of-pocket charges or the withdrawal of exemptions at the point of use are resisted by the French clectorate

- Rationing healthcare benefits other than marginally is unacceptable in France

Supplementary insurance cover has increasingly been used as a cushion between the crisis in national health insurance and the public's dislike of being uninsured at the point of use. It has enabled the state to transfer part of its financial burden to the *mutuelles* and private insurers. The public, for its part, has shown a clear preference

for paying supplementary insurance premiums rather than unrecoverable cash. This compromise has hitherto preserved the most characteristic features of French health care: its lavish offer, its freedom of choice, its high quality and generally good standard of outcomes, its organisational inefficiency, and its popularity with a grateful public.
  The facts:

• Supplementary health insurance pays for benefits that are not covered by *Assurance-Maladie*

• 84 per cent of the French population have a supplementary health insurance policy (compared with about one-third in 1960 and half in 1970)

• In 1998, about three-quarters of all supplementary insurance policies were taken out by individuals (including voluntary policies *via* their employers), and one-quarter were obligatory under the terms of employment

• There are three types of supplementary insurers: non-profit mutual societies (*mutuelles*), private insurers, and providence societies (*institutions de prévoyance*), jointly managed by employers and unions: the three types of insurers represented approximately 62 per cent, 22 per cent and 16 per cent of beneficiaries, respectively, in 1998.

(Source: CREDES Survey[20])

  In 1996, supplementary insurers financed the following percentages of French health care:

Table 2.5.1
Supplementary Insurance: % of Healthcare Finance, 1996

Insurer	Hospitals	Ambulatory Care	Pharma & Prostheses	TOTAL health care
Mutuelles	2.3	11.1	13.0	7.0
Private	0.9	5.3	5.4	3.1
Prévoyance	0.5	2.8	3.3	1.7
TOTAL	3.7	19.2	21.7	11.8

Source: Ministère de l'Emploi et de la Solidarité.[21]

  With supplementary insurers responsible for 11.8 per cent of French healthcare expenditure and private households for an additional 13.8 per cent, the state is relieved of over one-quarter of all health spending. The hospital sector is least affected, with 90 per cent coverage by the public sector.

Contrary to a widely held view, supplementary insurance has not raised French consumption appreciably. An analysis of ambulatory care (19 per cent covered by supplementary insurers) between 1980 and 1991 demonstrated that its growth was responsible for 0.3 percentage points out of a total annual growth rate of 2.4 per cent. This was partly because increased supplementary insurance is to some extent linked with reduced public sector coverage.[22]

The cost of supplementary insurance in France, with almost universal participation by the population and its limited impact on consumption, seems a price worth paying as a workable alternative to healthcare rationing.

6

Germany: *Achtung!* Rationing Alert!

Die derzeitige Gesundheitspolitik versucht einmal mehr, Probleme von gestern mit den Mitteln von vorgestern zu lösen.

The present health policy is trying once again to solve yesterday's problems with methods of the day-before-yesterday.

Dieter Cassel[1]

The German healthcare system of social insurance was the first to adopt the solidarity principle whereby society will take financial responsibility for the health care of those who are unable to look after themselves. As elsewhere in Europe, this noble principle was stretched during the twentieth century until it began to mean that nearly everyone would receive nearly everything in health care free (or nearly free) at the point of use. By the end of the century, social insurance in Germany—as in France, and like tax-based insurance in the UK—was chronically under threat of financial imbalance.

German health care is less centralised than the French system, but subject to federal rules and norms which all of the many sickness funds (*Krankenkassen*) must observe. In addition, capital expenditure for hospitals (but not their operating costs) is the responsibility of the states (*Länder*) of the Federal Republic. Apart from a small segment of private insurance, the German system is regarded as publicly financed irrespective of who actually owns the *Krankenkassen* who are the main insurers and payers.

Public expenditure on health in Germany in 1998 was 75 per cent of total expenditure, compared with 76 per cent in France and 84 per cent in the UK. Total spending per head of population in $PPP (purchasing power parities) was 2,424 compared with 2,077 in France and 1,461 in the UK (*OECD Health Data 2000*).

There is common ground between the German and French systems: both have high levels of expenditure by international standards, lavish provision with surplus capacity of medical facilities and services, relatively inefficient organisational performance, and a high degree of public satisfaction (although by many outcome measures, France achieves better results). This contrasts with the UK's low expenditure commitment, shortages, fairly high levels of efficiency relative to resources, often poor outcomes, and uncertain (probably declining) public satisfaction (see Part II-1, 2, 3).

The German Battle For Cost Containment

During the past 20 years, despite Germany's market economy, health care has been increasingly subjected not just to medical regulation but to strenuous financial control in the name of cost containment.

The root cause, as in France, is that the system can no longer respond to demand by raising employers' and employees' health insurance contributions. The *Krankenkassen* have a statutory duty to balance their books. For decades, they were able to do this by raising premiums. In Germany, these are based on gross wages and salaries up to a salary ceiling beyond which no further payment is required and the insured can opt out of the GKV (*Gesetzliche Krankenversicherung* —Statutory Health Insurance).

Premiums have risen from about eight per cent in the late-1970s to 13.5 per cent in mid-1998 (13.9 per cent in the former East Germany). They are shared equally between employer and employed.

Die GKV leidet ... weniger unter einem Ausgaben- als unter einem Einnahme-problem.

The problem of Statutory Health Insurance is not so much its outgoings as its income.[2]

This income problem, referred to in the quotation, is characteristic of employer-based social insurance systems during periods of low economic growth. During most of the 1990s, the German economy was sluggish, aggravated by the parlous state of the former East Germany. Unemployment was high, wages and salaries were stable, and the GKV's increasingly painful income problem had to confront steadily rising demand for health care which is largely independent of national economic performance.

By this time, employers were strongly resisting further increases in health insurance premiums, claiming that the high level of social charges was making German industry internationally uncompetitive.

Growing confrontation between industry and health care forced government to make choices. The validity of the assertion that the rising cost of employers' health insurance payments is destroying competitiveness has been disputed both in Germany and in the USA (where a similar problem has arisen between employers and managed care). The magnitude of the damage done to industry certainly leaves room for argument. *Politically*, however, German fears in the mid-1990s of a progressive de-industrialisation of the country lent strong support to policies that would uphold *Standort Deutschland*—the choice of Germany for investment and industrial development. As a result, the emphasis in health care was changed decisively from higher premiums in response to rising consumption, to stable contributions and more rigorous cost containment.

Competition With Velvet Paws

One aspect of this new policy during the 1990s has been legislative reform introducing some degree of competition between sickness funds; for example, reform has made it possible for patients to change their sickness fund without notice when premiums are raised and better terms can be obtained elsewhere.

The main result of pressure to compete has, paradoxically, been to narrow the disparities in premiums offered by different *Krankenkassen* and to encourage mergers which have materially reduced the number of sickness funds in Germany.

The drive to develop a competitive healthcare system in Germany is half-hearted and cannot be compared with the competitive climate in US health care. Basically, German sickness funds can compete only on premiums and the quality of their reputation (or their reputation for quality care). Their *product* offer is federally standardised. Changing it or offering packages of specific healthcare goods and services at differential prices is prohibited by law; nor can sickness funds bargain individually with individual physicians, hospitals or suppliers. The system is run as an organised duopoly of the Leading Associations of Sickness Funds (*Spitzenverbände der Krankenkassen*) and the Federal Association of Sickness Fund Physicians (*Kassenärztliche Bundesverei-nigung*) who negotiate collectively.[3] The power that springs from this arrangement favours a relatively uncompetitive *status quo*.

Although market forces operate in German health care to the extent that prices are not controlled, competition is at best hesitant and muted. Consequently, public policy has focused more and more desperately on cost containment.

'Efficiency Reserves'

A prominent aim of public policy has been to achieve substantial savings by drawing on the system's 'efficiency reserves' (*Ausschöpfung der Wirtschaftlichkeitsreserven*)—in other words, to run the system more efficiently, for which there was ample scope. The Advisory Council for Concerted Action (*Konzertierte Aktion*), in a report commissioned by the then Health Minister, pointed out that:

> The excess number of hospital beds, doctors, pharmacies, pharmaceuticals and medical technology are examples of one type of efficiency reserve. Excess capacity does not only provide incentives for the provision of unnecessary care, sometimes even with adverse medical effects, but also removes resources from other part of the healthcare system and in the general economy. (Advisory Council for Concerted Action in Health Care, published English translation, 1996.)[4]

This strategy has predictably run into the difficulty encountered by all healthcare policies that are based primarily or solely on efficiency targets: after making the easy savings, further progress is slow and begins to meet ferocious resistance from vested interests.

The 'inefficiency' of the German healthcare system is only partly operational and organisational. These are the areas where improvements can be achieved without a political backlash. In reality, inefficiency is above all structural: there is a large surplus of doctors (even larger than in France) and of hospital capacity.

In Germany, there is no *numerus clausus* for medical students as in France, because the German constitution guarantees the right to medical education subject only to entrance qualifications. Instead, the authorities have tried to stop settlement of new doctors with allocation procedures in areas where there is already a substantial surplus.[5]

The rationalisation of hospital capacity has proven even more difficult because hospital facilities are a *Länder* responsibility, whereas operating costs are borne by the GKV. Regional authorities are well aware of the extreme electoral unpopularity of local hospital closures and the main result is deadlock.

The lack of progress of radical changes designed to release 'efficiency reserves' has intensified the drive to extract savings from easier targets: the doctors and the pharmaceutical industry. It is these initiatives that have taken parts of the healthcare system beyond normal cost containment into the grey area and have set the alarm bells ringing: '*Achtung!* Rationing is on the way!'.

The warning raises the intriguing question: is it gesture politics or is Germany really in for healthcare rationing?

1999: The Summer Of Discontent

For more than 20 years, cost containment initiatives have ruled German health policy. More than a dozen legislative initiatives produced nothing more than temporary expenditure cuts and have therefore always set off new measures. (author's translation)[6]

These measures ranged at first from expenditure targets and the introduction of modest user charges, to the more recent reference prices for drugs (*Festbeträge*), and sectoral budgets with capped expenditure for hospitals, physicians, pharmaceuticals and dental care, as well as more substantial increases in user charges.

Capped budgets for doctors in ambulatory care introduced a serious conflict of interest. If expenditure exceeds the capped sum, collective penalty payments by the profession would directly affect physicians' incomes. In that event, would doctors downgrade pharmaceutical prescribing in order to avert the risk of deductions from their personal incomes?

Here, anecdotal and statistical evidence differ. Stories and individual testimony point to *some* doctors fobbing off their more docile patients with cheap products when a costly innovative prescription drug would have been better medicine. Some doctors have also proposed operations ('not on my budget') when drug therapy ('on my budget') would have been at least as effective and a considerably cheaper form of health care than surgery. Numerous such examples were cited in November 1999 in an article entitled *'Teure Patienten unerwünscht'* ('Expensive patients unwelcome') in *Die Zeit*.[7]

Collectively, on the other hand, German doctors have continued to look for 'efficiency reserves' whilst prescribing responsibly for the majority of patients. Annual analyses of prescribing patterns in the GKV market have consistently shown a decline in the so-called *Umstrittene Arzneimittel* (drugs of disputed medical value) from a peak of about 750 million prescriptions in 1992 to less than half that number in 1998. In that year, prescriptions of these 'disputed' drugs fell by 6.7 per cent while drug prescriptions as a whole fell only by 3.2 per cent. By contrast, new and innovative drugs continued to advance, and cheap generics increased their market share in competition with brands in the unpatented segment of the market.[8]

Whilst the trend in savings on 'disputed' drugs and generics has not been large enough to counterbalance the 'structural' impact on expenditure of new drugs, there has evidently been no general decline in the standard of prescribing by German doctors in spite of the threat of penalty payments.

Instead, there have been panic moves towards rationing by the KBV (*Kassenärztliche Bundesvereinigung* – Federal Association of Sickness Fund Physicians) which represents the medical profession in the GKV. In the summer of 1999, the KBV observed that only three of the 23 doctors' associations (KVs) were likely to keep within their drug budgets for the calendar year. In order not to trigger penalty payments, the KBV devised an Emergency Programme which would, in effect, ration drug prescribing for the rest of the year.[9]

The Emergency Programme proposed five steps:

1. Waiting lists for prescription drugs and other prescription treatments (*Heilmittel*, which include physiotherapy, acupuncture etc.) except in life threatening or medically essential circumstances

2. Postponement of innovative therapy to the following budget year

3. Radical switching of prescriptions from brand to the *cheapest* generic

4. Prior authorisation of expensive therapies

5. In the event of budget being exceeded, 'emergency prescriptions' to

be issued temporarily, for which patients would have to pay out-of-pocket and personally claim reimbursement (in Germany, unlike France, patients pay only user charges out of pocket)

This programme was clearly a full-blooded form of rationing as defined by the criteria set out in Part I-3 of this study:

The first criterion, *scarcity of physical resources*, was fulfilled in an artificial and bureaucratic rather than a real manner: prescriptions were viewed in the programme *as though* drugs and other treatments were not available, because doctors would risk losing income as a result of behaving like doctors.

The second element of rationing, *waiting lists*, was directly included in the emergency programme (point 1).

The third element, *denial of quality treatment*, was explicitly covered by point 2, and implied in point 4 of the proposals.

The fourth aspect, *discrimination between patients regardless of need*, was embodied in point 5 and risked occurring as a result of points 1 and 4.

The Emergency Programme had a tumultuous reception. One commentator, after noting that antidiarrhoeal drugs were to be wait-listed, enquired sarcastically whether treatment of 'acute diarrhoea was to be postponed until next year while the waiting list was being systematically run down?'[10]

The Ministry of Health dismissed the programme as unnecessary and absurd, and threatened government intervention if the KBV persisted in pursuing it. There was a mixed reaction from various organisations of doctors, some hostile, some silently neutral, others supporting the move as a form of protest against government policies. The sickness funds protested, as did the research-based pharmaceutical industry.[11]

This was not the first occasion when the Federal Association of Sickness Fund Doctors has proposed emergency rationing. There was a previous and similar proposal in 1996 which was never activated. Was the 1999 initiative simply a political stunt for the silly season of the summer holidays, or was it meant to be taken seriously?

The answer appeared to be: *both*, for the abandonment of the Emergency Programme as such was swiftly followed by a Joint Action Programme agreed between the KBV on behalf of the doctors, the Federal Association of the *Krankenkassen* on behalf of the insurers, and the Federal Ministry of Health.

The Joint Action Programme 1999

The objective of this programme was to ensure that the 1999 drug and *Heilmittel* budgets would be adhered to. It consisted of nine points:

1. Basis and realisation of the programme

2. Prescription of generics at prices within the lowest third of the range

3. Negative list of 'trivial' medicines

4. Exclusion of anabolics and vitamin combination products

5. Reimbursable prescribing of certain listed drugs in accordance with official Medicines Guidelines only after non-medicinal alternatives have been tried first and have failed

6. Avoidance of 'disputed' medicines (*Umstrittene Arzneimittel*)

7. Avoidance of expensive innovative improvements (*Schrittinnovationen*) 'of uncertain added value in terms of therapeutic utility'

8. Prior authorisation before prescribing a list of drugs involving 'expensive therapy which might, in particular cases, be of disputed or minimal therapeutic benefit'

9. Measures for ensuring that only 'medically necessary' *Heilmittel* are prescribed[12]

The urgency of the Joint Action Programme was emphasised by letters from local Associations of Sickness Funds Doctors to their GPs, of which the following extract represents the mixed ingredients of appeal and threat:

Sehr geehrte Kolleginnen und Kollegen, nur die konsequente Umsetzung der 'Massnahmen des Aktionsprogramms' kann noch verhindern, dass es im Jahre 1999 auch im KV-Bereich 'X' zu einer Budgetüberschreitung und damit zu pauschalen Regressforderungen kommt. Deshalb appellieren wir nochmals sehr eindringlich an Sie, sich diesem Aktionsprogramm nicht zu verschliessen.

Dear Colleagues, Only the determined pursuit of the 'Measures of the Action Programme' can still prevent the budget for 1999 being exceeded and proportionate penalty payments being demanded in the area of this Association. That is why we appeal to you once more and most emphatically not to ignore this Action Programme.

The letter was accompanied by an information sheet making it clear to 'difficult' and demanding patients that they have no right to claim anything beyond 'medically necessary' medicines but that 'your doctor ...can if you wish give you a private prescription. Your *Krankenkasse* is not allowed to reimburse it'. That will soon teach those who, like Oliver Twist, ask for more.

It is worth examining whether this Joint Action Programme, whilst far less radical than the original proposals of the KBV, also contains elements of rationing. Whereas the purpose of the Action Programme was purely budgetary for 1999, it clearly implies prescribing practices that could equally be invoked for the management of physician's budgets in subsequent years. Taking the four rationing criteria in turn:

1. *Scarcity of physical resources* is neither claimed nor implied in the nine-point Action Programme. The only resource that is in short supply is money until the end of the financial year. In terms of resources, the measures are intended to fulfil the classic purpose of cost containment, not to ration supply.

2. *Waiting lists* are not included or intended, although point 8 (prior authorisation) could in practice involve delays.

3. *Denial of quality treatment* is a possibility in points 7 and 8, and conceivable (though relatively unlikely) in relation to the drug classes that are listed in point 5. The word 'expensive'—one of the signals when quality is to be rationed—is used in both 7 and 8.

The question of including or excluding 'innovative improvements' from reimbursement has been controversial throughout the last twenty years. Medical practice suggests that patients are individual in their response to many categories of drugs: what suits one may cause serious side reactions in another. There should always be room for drug improvements in the rules for reimbursement. Payers, on the other hand, believe that innovative improvements are too expensive and should therefore be avoided (as in the Action Programme) or excluded. This view seems unwise and short-sighted, because it can lead to distortions in prescribing towards either less effective or even more expensive drugs that are not on the 'avoidance' list.

Obtaining a second opinion (*Zweitmeinung,* point 8) may be fully justified if it is for medical reasons alone. Once the word *expensive* creeps into the description of a drug, the procedure lies in the grey area between cost containment and rationing. The second opinion has become prior authorisation and the decision maker is an official of the payer, who maybe medically qualified but whose objectives are primarily financial. Delay and denial of quality then become distinct possibilities.

4. *Discrimination between patients regardless of need* is implied by several points on the Action Programme. Point 3 ('trivial' medicines) discriminates between patients under the age of 18 (for whom reimbursement of such products is allowed) and older patients. The definition of 'triviality' includes cough and cold medicines, mouth and throat products, and travel sickness remedies.

Points 5, 6, 7 and 8 all present similarly ambivalent possibilities of putting the budget ahead of the patient's needs. To prescribe a listed drug only after non-medicinal alternatives have been tried and failed can be regarded as sound common sense; it can also be viewed as allowing need to be disregarded for budgetary reasons and giving the right treatment too late.

The avoidance of 'disputed' medicines (point 6) sounds perfectly reasonable, but also puts the budget ahead of the patient. 'Disputed' medicines are the subject of dispute: they have not been proven either effective or ineffective. Many patients appear to derive benefit from them and many doctors regard the *placebo* effect as a relatively inexpensive way of dealing with the problems of some patients. That is not a defence of 'disputed' medicines, but merely a recognition, in Hamlet's words, that 'there are more things in heaven and earth than are dreamt of in your philosophy'. When the patient, rather than the budget, comes first, there is sometimes room for giving the disputed medicine the benefit of the doubt.

The possibilities of discrimination between patients over point 7 ('innovative improvements') and 8 (prior authorisation), as already discussed above, are evidently considerable.

In the light of the above analysis, the Joint Action Programme cannot be described as an outright instrument of rationing, but its penetration into the grey area at several points is undeniable. It is a compromise between the traditional freedom of choice on the part of German doctors and patients, and the rationing principle. One could describe it as a form of 'proto-rationing': *Achtung!* You never know what's round the corner.

The Rump Reform Of 1999-2000

Looked at from a rationing point of view, the Schröder Administration's reform bill of 1999 was a step in the wrong direction. The administration had already reversed previous measures to increase user charges, although the reductions were modest enough to count as political gestures rather than as serious instruments of policy. Evidently, higher user charges will help to stave off rationing by transferring some payments from the state to the patient.

In the summer of 1999, Health Minister Andrea Fischer promised 'stable GKV contributions' as the cornerstone of her reform. A global capped budget for health care was to be the main tool for achieving stable premiums.[13] This would cap hospital, ambulatory, pharmaceutical and other medical expenditure, again requiring penalty payments from doctors in the event of excess. It was also to introduce a 'positive list' for prescription drugs which meant that only listed products would be reimbursed.

The reform proposals ran into trouble when it became clear that the upper house (*Bundesrat*) of the German parliament, in which the ruling coalition does not have a majority, would reject it. As a result, a compromise 'rump' reform which included only items that did not require approval by the upper house, was negotiated in conference between the two chambers. To achieve this, the proposals had to be watered down by excluding the 'global budget', the positive list for drugs, and the reform of hospital finance.[14]

Whether this has changed the 'proto-rationing' climate in Germany is doubtful. Although the 'global budget' principle with its collective responsibility for not exceeding the expenditure cap had to be sacrificed, this merely signals a return to the old and relatively unsuccessful principle of sectoral budgets, with the expectation that these will be tightened. Moreover, the abandonment of radical changes in hospital finance means that the structural problems of controlling hospital expenditure and extracting the long-sought 'efficiency reserves' will continue in abeyance.

What The Public Thinks Of The GKV (Statutory Health Insurance)

In December 1999, WIdO (the Scientific Institute of the AOK, the largest grouping of sickness funds) published a survey[15] of about 3,000 German households, conducted in the spring of 1998 and the spring of 1999. They were asked what they expected the GKV to offer in the way of health care.

Among the many questions and answers, those that are relevant to the themes of this report are discussed below. All responses were measured on a five-point scale, for example: 'Agree totally, agree on the whole, neither agree nor disagree, disagree on the whole, disagree totally'. For the purpose of this report, the sum of the two most negative responses has been deducted from the sum of the two most positive ones (ignoring the 'neither/nors', 'don't knows' and 'others') to give a net plus or net minus result measured in percentage points.

The German public is overwhelmingly satisfied with the services offered by their own *Krankenkasse* (+77.5 per cent points). In an 'ideal' *Krankenkasse,* the highest importance (4.5-4.6 marks out of five) was assigned to 'generous' benefits, rapid and unbureaucratic assistance, competent advisers, and a complete range of services. Respondents gave their own *Krankenkasse* marks that fell short of perfection but were well above average (=2.5): generous benefits 3.8, rapid assistance 4.0, complete range of services 4.0, competent advisers 4.1.

Rationing would, by definition, hit at least three of these top-*desiderata*: benefits would become less generous, assistance more bureaucratic and probably slower, and the range of services would be less complete.

Interestingly, when asked to comment on the statement that 'the solidarity principle is no longer appropriate in today's society', 22.3 per cent agreed and 47.0 per cent disagreed: net result only 24.7 per cent points in favour of solidarity, while just over 30 per cent could not decide. This suggests that rationing in the name of solidarity might still have limited but no longer whole-hearted support. The consequences of rationing would adversely affect the comparison between the respondent's own *Krankenkasse* with what an ideal sickness fund should be offering. That could well create considerable discontent before long.

Despite Germany's market economy, respondents overwhelmingly favoured more controls: pharmaceutical price control (+81.7 per cent points); control of treatment quality in ambulatory and institutional care (+65.1 per cent); and controlling whether the work of doctors and hospitals is *wirtschaftlich* (economic or cost-effective) (+53.4 per cent).

It is difficult to know what to make of these preferences for the mechanisms of control. Probably, they are part of the central theme of German healthcare policy: no more increases in contributions. 'Controlling' healthcare goods and services—in other words, controlling costs—must be 'a good thing' if it helps to achieve the goal of stable contributions; better, in any event, than making *me* pay more.

These responses about controls are part of the 'leading question' syndrome that will produce predictable or politically correct answers (see Part I-3). They are not a particularly sound guide to actual political decisions, because respondents ignore the consequences of control.

The overall conclusions of the survey are that those who demand fundamental reforms, including 'more market' or 'steps to ration benefits' in the GKV 'must produce sound reasons'.[16]

With a population that is evidently highly satisfied with the existing system, such a conclusion is not surprising. Nevertheless, there will be sound reasons for and even sounder reasons against rationing health care in Germany.

Conclusions

Although threats and accusations of rationing are being bandied about in German healthcare politics, the evidence suggests that current practices and reforms of the system do *not* amount to rationing.

Of the principal criteria:

There is no physical scarcity of resources as a general rule. Waiting lists are not endemic but exceptional. Denial of quality treatment and discrimination between patients are, however, creeping into the system, often by what is being referred to as 'invisible rationing'. The intention is not to deny or to discriminate, but increasingly restrictive legislation and controls are 'hidden persuaders' in how physicians and institutions might be able to cut a corner or two. The grey area between cost containment and rationing is becoming larger and, in places, visible. '*Achtung!* Rationing Alert!' seems to be a slogan that fits the situation.

On these grounds, Germany scores less well than France though much better than the UK.

7

The USA: The Power to Make Choices

The choice is between imperfect government and imperfect market; the political process is biased towards advocating government as a solution for market problems rather than markets as a solution for governmental problems; and the power to make choices is the power to make mistakes.

Mark V. Pauly[1]

Public and private health care in the USA can no longer be classed as entirely separate. Most patients in public sector schemes also have private health insurance: among Medicare beneficiaries in 1995, only eight per cent had no form of supplementary health insurance; 19 per cent had additional public sector coverage; and 62 per cent had employer-sponsored or individually purchased private insurance. The remaining 11 per cent were not identified by source of funds.[2]

Increasing numbers of public sector patients have also enrolled with managed care organisations (MCOs), voluntarily or by state mandate. Managed care, despite its problems and faults, is probably the most influential American contribution to the running of private as well as public sector health care in the closing decades of the twentieth century.

To this, many European commentators would reply: 'But we have been "managing" care long before America did—ever since 1945 or even earlier!' True; but not competitively. Most of Europe is run by single-payer economic and financial regulation, with scarcely a nod in the direction of market forces. Financially, health care in Europe is centrally or regionally *controlled*, not 'managed'. In the USA, only the public sector is under federal or state financial control, but even there the iron grip has been sufficiently relaxed to let private sector MCOs *manage* care on behalf of public sector bodies.

The private sector as a whole is responsible for a little over half of all healthcare expenditure in the USA.

The Vexed Question Of Access

America is bursting with Americans who are critical of America's healthcare system or systems or lack of system. The healthcare scene is a patchwork of infinite complexity, variety and flexibility. It produces the best and the worst healthcare conditions side by side. Its long-standing problem has *not* been the battle between control and market forces, or between cost and quality, but between access and lack of access: the question of equity.

In the context of this study, it is as well to state at the outset that inequality of access is *not* rationing. Rationing is the mechanism of distributing scarce resources. There is no scarcity in the land of plenty. There is no perceptible urge to *allocate* which is the substance of rationing. What is absent in the USA is an overriding sense of solidarity which is the bedrock of European health care. The USA is still imbued with the pioneering virtues of personal responsibility and self-help which solidarity has submerged in Europe. That is an observation, not a recommendation, nor a condemnation. The most that American health care has until now been willing to concede to solidarity is universal (though imperfect) access for the old and disabled, and the provision of 'welfare' health care for the poor.

The notorious 44 million Americans (16 per cent of the population) who are uninsured are left out by the nation's *non*-system. They can receive free emergency treatment but are largely deprived of 'normal' health care. The core of the uninsured are the so-called 'near-poor' or 'working poor' who are not sufficiently well-off to take out private insurance, are not covered by their employers, and are not poor enough to qualify for public sector Medicaid. On either side of this poverty trap are those who can afford health insurance but decide not to buy it, and those who are entitled to public assistance but fail to claim it. The latter run into millions. In 1998, a federal estimate concluded that about 4.7 million children were uninsured although eligible for Medicaid:

> The number of people who are not taking advantage of Medicaid coverage is quite large, and the problem speaks of the obstacles that many poor people face in trying to navigate publicly run systems.[3]

The Public/Private Mix: Facts

In 1960, public funds accounted for only 24.5 per cent of total national health expenditure in the USA. By 1970, this had risen to 37.8 per cent, mainly as a result of the setting up of Medicare and Medicaid by the Johnson Administration in 1965, as part of that President's 'Great Society' policy. It was America's largest leap towards solidarity in the twentieth century. All previous and subsequent attempts to adopt universal coverage, from the Roosevelt and Truman Administrations to that of President Clinton, have been either aborted or defeated in Congress.

Nevertheless, Congress has voted for a series of smaller steps at intervals ever since the 1960s. By 1985, public funds were responsible for 40.6 per cent of national health expenditure, and by 1997 this had risen further to its highest level yet, 46.2 per cent, decreasing slightly to 45.5 per cent in 1998.[4]

The Health Care Financing Administration (HCFA) estimates that there will be modest falls from the 1997 peak to 44.8 per cent in 2001-2 and a reversion to 46.4 per cent by 2008 (www.hcfa.gov/stats/nhe-proj, update 12 July 1999).

The main explanation for the rise in the public share of health spending in recent years is the cost containment impact of managed care on private expenditure. The latter rose only by 9.9 per cent *per capita* between 1993 and 1997, whereas public *per capita* expenditure increased by 26.9 per cent over the same period (web site, as above). This trend slowed in 1998 and may come to a halt temporarily, because managed care has already extracted the easy savings from the private sector, and because private insurance premiums are rising again.

In reality, the USA now has a mixed private/public healthcare economy in which the two sectors are almost evenly matched in terms of spending. As noted in Part II-1, health care in the USA ranks 4th among 29 OECD member states in *public* expenditure per head of population and 12th in *public* spending as a percentage of Gross Domestic Product.

The structure of the public/private expenditure mix in 1998 was as follows:

Table 2.7.1
USA National Health Expenditure, % by Source of Funds, 1998

	%	%
Private health insurance	32.6	
Patients out-of-pocket	17.4	
Other private	4.5	
Total private		54.5
Federal (of which Medicare 18.8)	32.8	
State and local	12.7	
Total public (of which Medicaid 14.8)		45.5
		100

Source: Levit, Cowan, Lazenby *et al*. [5]

Between 1993 and 1997, private insurance and patients' out-of-pocket payments fell as a proportion of total healthcare spending, whereas Medicaid (which receives federal and state funds) and particularly Medicare (federally funded) rose. Except for Medicaid, these trends reversed in 1998.

Public/private expenditure ratios differ materially in various healthcare sectors:

Table 2.7.2
USA: % Sources of Funds in Different Healthcare Sectors, 1997

Sector	Public	Private	Total
	%	%	%
Hospitals	61.6	38.4	100
Nursing homes	62.2	37.8	100
Physician services	32.2	67.8	100
Prescription drugs	20.2	79.8	100
Dental services	4.3	95.7	100

Source: Braden, Cowan et al.[6]

Whereas over 60 per cent of hospital and nursing home expenditure came from public funds, the public share for physicians was less than one-third, and for pharmaceuticals only one-fifth. Dental services are almost entirely privately paid for.

Medicare and Medicaid

Medicare is a programme for seniors (65+), the disabled, and for patients with end stage renal disease (ESRD—kidney failure). Part A of Medicare covers hospital and related care, and is funded from payroll taxes that are shared equally by employer and employee. In addition, there is cost sharing by beneficiaries when they receive treatment. Part B covers physician and outpatient (and related) services and is financed from general taxation and from premiums payable by beneficiaries.[7]

Medicaid is a programme for persons with low incomes, including the elderly and disabled (who can also enrol in Medicare), and those receiving public assistance. It is financed by federal and state funds in varying proportions. The federal share can range from 50 per cent to 83 per cent.

The most important difference between the two programmes is that Medicare provides *universal* federal coverage for all seniors, whereas Medicaid resembles (and is regarded as) a welfare service. For Medicaid, each of the states 'set their own standards of eligibility; determine the type, amount, duration and scope of covered services; establish the rate of payment for services; and administer their own programs'.[8] The distinction has meant that Medicare is prized by the public because all who qualify have a *right* to it, whilst Medicaid is tainted by the welfare image. That is made worse by the fact that applicants for Medicaid have to be tested for eligibility before they are accepted or rejected.

Federally, the HCFA is responsible for both Medicare and Medicaid. The HCFA sets out basic rules which the administrators of both prog- rammes are obliged to respect. These include certain mandatory services and benefits, leaving the states to offer additional, optional benefits at their discretion. Reimbursement and provider fees, too, are subject to HCFA's framework rules and requirements.

Another important difference between Medicare and Medicaid is that, under existing rules, Medicare does not provide out-patient drug benefit (with a few exceptions for self-administered infusions), whereas Medicaid programmes can reimburse prescription drugs in accordance with HCFA rules going back to 1976. Plans to include a drug benefit in Medicare have been controversial for years and are again under discussion in Congress at this time.

In 1998, the total cost of Medicare was $217 billion and Medicaid $171billion. There were 38.8 million Medicare beneficiaries (14 per cent of the US population) and 41.3 million (in 1997) were eligible for Medicaid (15 per cent of the population). Twenty-six per cent of Medicaid recipients are seniors or disabled, and may be in both programmes.

Altogether, approximately 25 per cent of the US population are covered by the public sector, including Medicare, Medicaid, the Department of Defence, the Veterans Administration and others. With nearly half of US healthcare expenditure attributable to the public sector, and its rapid rate of growth, it is not surprising that cost containment is high on the political agenda.

Is The Public Sector Containing Costs Or Rationing Health Care?

Most of the literature on the subject, and most Americans with whom the author has discussed it, agree that there is little overt rationing in US public sector health care. There are exceptions, like organ grafts of which there is a shortage in the USA as elsewhere (see Part I-4) and the Oregon experiment (discussed below). There is also a wide grey area that defies precise categorisation but may be epitomised as *veiled, implicit or silent* variants of rationing.

Even though access to Medicare is universal for seniors and the disabled, access to particular forms of treatment may be restricted. They may be time-limited (nursing care: 100 days after discharge from an acute care hospital); quality-reduced (hip replacement with a cheap but less durable prosthesis); or expenditure-capped (rehabilitation speech therapy up to $1,500). In Medicaid, drug treatment may be volume-capped (number of tablets, or prescriptions, or refills in a given time period) or excluded from closed prescription drug formularies. Prior authorisation of interventions or prescriptions exists in both programmes.

The grey area is defined by restricted budgets. Public funds for health care remain a highly controversial topic in Congress, with powerful lobbies resisting the spread of 'solidarity'. On the other hand, the inclusion of ESRD patients in Medicare since 1973 was a step towards equal access in the one major area where physical shortages, waiting lists and rationing are the rule (see Part I-4). In 1999, 86 per cent of all ESRD patients in the USA were covered by public funds (80 per cent by Medicare), about ten per cent by private insurance, and four per cent were uninsured or paid out-of-pocket.[9] Here, public funds have reduced the hardship that the majority of ESRD patients would have had to endure from lack of access even to the rationing process for otherwise unaffordable treatment. While waiting lists for organ grafts continue, Medicare has effectively ended the rationing of kidney dialysis:

> Previously, dialysis had been rationed and deferred via waiting lists ... patients were dying, not because there was no effective treatment but because of budget constraints and the resulting limited supply of dialysis machines.[10]

The main emphasis in Medicare cost containment is on pricing (especially of hospital and physician fees), not on rationing of patients' benefits. Capitated fees began to replace *per diem* hospital charges in the 1980s with the introduction of the prospective payment system and the adoption of diagnosis-related groups (DRGs) for the classification of patients. Similarly, payment of physicians moved progressively from fee-for-service to relative value units (based on time and complexity of services performed), which were officially adopted by the HCFA in 1991.[11]

Medicare must offer quality health care to beneficiaries who, it is estimated, are paying approximately 30 per cent of the total cost of their treatment under Medicare: 23 per cent by cost-sharing in Part A and premiums for Part B, and about seven per cent for acute care services that Medicare does not cover.[12]

Medicaid, by contrast, has moved rather further into the grey area between cost containment and rationing. The blend between federal and state funding is, in a sense, a contest about which side can get away with spending less. The welfare tinge of Medicaid, too, puts limits to what state politicians are prepared to allow in budgeting for Medicaid expenditure.

Although Medicaid has unquestionably been successful in improving access by the poor to general health services, it has been much less successful in ensuring access to mainstream care. Private physicians did not respond to the program as its architects had assumed they would ... Over 25 per cent of the nation's private practice physicians do not accept Medicaid patients.[13]

For pharmaceuticals, HCFA rules define maximum allowable cost (MAC) or similar limits for drug prices. In addition, drug companies must offer Medicaid rebates of at least 15 per cent below average wholesale prices, or the 'best price' that is offered to any other US purchaser. Medicaid cannot actually exclude drugs that are 'medically necessary', but state programmes can define how such drugs are to be reimbursed and can also conduct lengthy negotiations about discounts with pharmaceutical companies before listing new drugs. Such delays, together with the design of formularies and rules for prior authorisation bring drug reimbursement by Medicaid into the grey area.

Among the 'tough' states is California, where negotiation to secure listing on the closed formulary of the state Medicaid organisation (Medi-Cal) can be a lengthy and difficult process:

A drug may be added to the list on contractual agreement by the manufacturer to provide the state a rebate based on the quantity reimbursed to pharmacies for Medi-Cal recipients. The patient's physician or pharmacist may request prior authorization from the field office Medi-Cal consultant for approval of unlisted drugs or for listed drugs that are restricted to specific use(s).[14]

Medi-Cal's limitations and exclusions are either for medical reasons (for example, restricted indications) or are the result of failure to obtain a large enough discount from a single-source supplier. These restrictions lie in the grey area. They cannot be described as outright rationing, because there is no shortage of supply; there are no waiting lists (compare the abortive waiting list proposals for drugs by the German physicians' association in Part II-6); the denial of quality treatment is usually limited to delay rather than absolute denial; and similarly, discrimination between patients can be averted if the physician is willing to go to the trouble of seeking prior authorisation— but many are not willing to do so.

A Congressional Hearing in 1993 discussed the question of whether state Medicaid formularies were a 'cost saving measure or second-class medicine'. The Louisiana Department of Health and Hospitals had abolished the state's restrictive formulary. Carolyn O. Maggio of that organisation testified that the state had decided in favour of a multi-source basis of reimbursement. This was limited to lower-cost drugs

... except where the physician certified a need for a specific drug brand in writing ... No prior authorization or bureaucratic red tape is required ... We have found that alternative approaches which support and supplement healthcare practitioners are more effective in containing costs than the development of bureaucratic processes.[15]

Whilst grey-area practices are found in many state Medicaid programmes, one state has committed its health plan to overt and explicit rationing: Oregon.

The Oregon Experiment

The Oregon experiment is famous worldwide for what is probably its least successful feature: the notorious cut-off list of reimbursable medical interventions for state Medicaid recipients:

> In 1991, Oregon ranked more than 700 diagnoses and treatments in order of importance. The state legislature then drew a line at item 587; treatments below the line would not be covered. Oregon had openly embraced the R-word: rationing—worse, rationing for the poor.[16]

'Rationing for the poor' was a slogan that opponents have consistently flung at the Oregon experiment which became operative in February 1994. The ranking list applied only to Medicaid recipients, not to Medicare beneficiaries or private patients. Yet the objective was worthy: the Oregon Health Plan tried to tackle America's most serious healthcare problem: its uninsured poor. Its main objective was to make all persons below the federal poverty level eligible for Medicaid by cutting out the complex eligibility criteria which lead to rejected applications or unwillingness to apply. In effect:

> All Oregonians with incomes under the federal poverty level ($13,000 for a family of three) are now eligible for Medicaid. Previously only 57 per cent of people with incomes under the poverty level were eligible.[17]

The additional cost had to be absorbed by savings in order to keep the Oregon Health Plan solvent. This was achieved in part by moving 87 per cent of enrollees into managed care, and in part by prioritising benefits and not reimbursing those below the dividing line.

The cut-off list of reimbursable benefits may with some justification be described as the apotheosis of prioritisation. For health experts, it is their wildest wish dream come true: the application of logical and democratic principles to the wonderful world of rationing.

To the innocent lay person, it is the latest version of Hans Christian Andersen's *The Emperor's New Clothes*. In the majestic procession of prioritised interventions, we are made to forget that it could all have been done in a much more rough-and-ready fashion by 'normal' cost containment methods, at a fraction of cost, effort, and pain, and without the accompaniment of international warfare between believers and unbelievers.

The results of Oregon's cut-off list have been trenchantly described:

[the cost-benefit principle] ...was effectively abandoned, partly because adequate data were lacking, partly because the exercise produced some counterintuitive results—for example, appendectomy ranked lower than tooth capping. The final rankings that appeared, after repeated massaging, seem to reflect judgments about 'reasonableness' taken in the light of community values. In other words, the attempt to apply clear-cut, transparent criteria was abandoned.[18]

Bodenheimer reported, however, that by the mid-1990s complaints about the list had more or less stopped. He attributed this to five reasons:

1. The plan as a whole has been applauded for having expanded health benefits

2. Most treatments below the cut-off line are recognised as relatively ineffective

3. Treatment below the line is often slipped in at the time of diagnosis, i.e. before the list can stop it. Sometimes there are 'complex diagnostic work-ups'(!)

4. Physicians 'game' the system by diagnosing 'above-the-line' illnesses for conditions that are listed 'below-the-line'

5. Direct activation of the list is only for the 13 per cent of Medicaid patients who consult fee-for-service physicians. 'But for the 87 per cent of Medicaid enrollees in capitated health plans, the state has shifted the financial risk to the plans and provides no additional funds if treatments listed below the line are given.'[19]

In other words, if one is trying to be a little too earnest and much too ingenious, doctors, patients and even the bureaucrats themselves will start playing games. It may be pertinent to observe that no other state has felt inclined to copy the Oregon experiment. However, in one respect the Oregon Health Plan is not unique: shifting the financial risk to managed care is a mainstream trend in both Medicaid and Medicare.

Medicare, Medicaid and Managed Care: A Loose Embrace

Romance?
Medicare loves Managed Care with unrequited passion. Managed Care is not sure whether it even likes Medicare. Medicaid and Managed Care are more comfortable in their embrace. Medicaid adores Managed Care who returns a measure of love as long as there is no interruption in the flow of dollars.

Medicare and Medicaid turned to managed care in the 1990s for the same reason that had motivated employer-based health insurance in the 1980s: energetic cost containment. There was a transfer of beneficiaries from mainly expensive fee-for-service health care to a mainly capitated system of fixed sums per member per month (PMPM). This reduced costs and helped budgetary control by shifting part or all of the financial risk to managed care. HCFA's healthcare rules and regulations for Medicare and Medicaid had also to be contractually observed by managed care organisations (MCOs).

Medicare patients were persuaded (not forced) to enrol in managed care with financial incentives, such as lower deductibles and/or lower co-payment. Another important incentive is that most MCOs offer drug benefit which Medicare does not cover for out-patients.

For Medicaid, the framework of transfers is different. The states can now require the mandatory transfer of Medicaid recipients to managed care, and about 40 states had done so by 1998. Until the early-1990s, it had been difficult for states to obtain HCFA waivers of the rules prohibiting mandatory transfer. The Clinton Administration encouraged the issuing of waivers and eventually abolished the need for such waivers altogether in the Balanced Budget Act of 1997.[20]

By 1997, over 50 per cent of Medicaid recipients were enrolled in managed care[21] compared with only 9.5 per cent in 1991. By contrast, the shift from fee-for-service to capitation in Medicare was far from a stampede: slower and much less intensive, it rose only from 4.8 per cent in 1990 to 13.9 per cent in 1997.[22] By 1998, the enrolment of Medicare patients in managed care had risen to about 17 per cent, but in 1999 it is estimated to have fallen back to 16 per cent, for reasons discussed below.

Whereas the majority of Medicaid recipients are obliged to transfer to managed care, Medicare beneficiaries can decide for themselves unless supplementary group insurers make the decision on their behalf. In 1995, as already stated, at least 62 per cent of Medicare beneficiaries also had private insurance (33 per cent employer-sponsored and 29 per cent individually purchased). More specifically, although Medicare provides virtually no out-patient drug coverage, nearly 50 per cent of Medicare beneficiaries had some form of third-party drug benefit.[23]

The incentives for Medicare beneficiaries to transfer to managed care are not pressing, and they are counter-balanced by a disinclination to being obliged to change family physicians as a result of transferring, for example, to a health maintenance organisation (HMO) with its own roster of physicians. There is also a fairly widespread fear that managed care may mean lower quality care. These misgivings were, however, eased by the Balanced Budget Act of 1997 which offered beneficiaries various forms of 'Medicare + Choice' that 'permit seniors to receive their health care from an expanded set of managed care options that go beyond the standard HMO option now available'.[24]

Managed Care: From Triumph To Backlash

As an instrument of cost containment, managed care seemed for some years to be the perfect answer to the problems of an employer-sponsored private health insurance system whose costs were out of control and escalating alarmingly. The public sector followed suit when it saw how successful managed care could be.

Managed care cut costs by the use of its bulk purchasing power; by tight budgetary management of expenditure; and by signing up hospitals and physicians under contracts that traded lower or capitated fees for a steady inflow of patients in a competitive system with ample spare capacity. Pharmaceutical expenditure was controlled by tough negotiations with manufacturers for large discounts from posted prices for single-source drugs as a condition of formulary listing; by prolific listing of cheap generics in place of brands unless the latter were also heavily discounted; and by imposing prescribing restrictions.

By 1996, about 43 per cent of all Americans had enrolled in managed care. By segment, 85 per cent of all *working* Americans and 77 per cent of private-sector employees were in managed care. In the public sector, as noted above, managed care had enrolled over 50 per cent of Medicaid recipients and 17 per cent of Medicare beneficiaries by 1998.

It seemed to be a *win-win* situation for all concerned. However, just when nearly everybody was responding to the cry of 'All Aboard!', the train began to move into the sidings for a quality check.

At first, it was mainly media stories of 'greedy' HMOs who, having 'picked the low-hanging fruit', were now pushing their luck and their bottom line at the expense of quality. Then the anecdotal sufferings of some managed care patients who had been denied expensive treatments to which they or their doctors believed they were entitled, made headlines in the media. Eventually, the backlash against managed care blew up into full-scale political warfare over a Patients' Bill of Rights, still unresolved in Congress at the time of writing.

These developments were probably inevitable. They are part and parcel of the 'efficiency delusion' discussed in Part II-4. It is common experience that, once the easier, genuine savings from greater efficiency have been achieved, further economy measures are often more apparent than real. The second phase of efficiency drives, in reality, is often an elaborate exercise in shifting burdens among the healthcare partners who 'are playing musical chairs in the hope of resolving the *political* question of Who Will Pay More or Receive Less when the music stops'.[25]

For managed care in the USA, the music stopped at least temporarily in the late-1990s. By 1998, HMOs had their third year of declining profits and actually registered a collective loss of $968 million.[26] HMOs tried to improve their low receipts from capitation in their 1999 Medicare contracts, but the HCFA turned down their requests. As a result, HMOs decided to increase user charges and reduce benefits. This, in effect, ejected those Medicare beneficiaries who were either unwilling or unable to pay more in return for less. It is believed to have reduced MCO enrolment from 17 per cent to 16 per cent of all Medicare beneficiaries in 1999. Some MCOs withdrew altogether from contracting with Medicare.

These reactions revealed some fundamental misconceptions by and about managed care. The initial period of glamour reflected managed care's skill in reducing the cost of health care for contracted groups of relatively healthy enrollees of working age whilst maintaining generally satisfactory standards of quality and of patient satisfaction. The transfer or adaptation of these management techniques to populations whose health is far less robust (seniors, the disabled, the poor and socially deprived) confronted the managers of MCOs with serious problems that were largely outside the range of experience that made managed care so successful. Congress, in turn, had imagined that managed care would manage Medicare and Medicaid patients with the same aplomb as patients with employer insurance, and the HCFA had imposed contractual terms which even for the more efficient MCOs were probably only marginally profitable. Excess capacity and competition did the rest: the world of managed care was increasingly in danger of becoming one of lower quality in order to achieve lower costs.

Managed Care, Competition, Innovation, And Rationing

Whatever doubts are being expressed about managed care, no one could accuse MCOs of failing to be competitive. It is their competitive drive for patients which at first prompted them to offer greater benefits at lower cost. When the down-cycle of competition eventually drove HMOs into the red, the up-cycle began by charging more for offering less, thereby driving the quality backlash into the arms of the lawmakers. Quality will be restored: either by competition or by law.

Apart from the more obvious direct forms of cost cutting, managed care has also been charged with reluctance to accept innovation (an important component of quality care) or even rationing its use. Pauly[27] has discussed the suggestion that managed care, more than traditional fee-for-service medicine, has targeted new technology because innovation drives spending. He concluded that the impact of managed care on technology remains an open question with conflicting evidence:

managed care has delayed the uptake of some technologies and rapidly accepted others. However, a dilemma is in the making:

> ...as managed care directly reduces the level of cost associated with old technology, such as fewer in-patient days, it will need to reduce the amount of new technology to a disproportionately greater extent to generate a lower growth in spending. Unless such a reduction can be made to occur, the slowdown in cost growth will be temporary rather than permanent.[28]

Experience in most healthcare systems in the industrialised world suggests that resistance to new technology, too, is temporary rather than permanent—above all, in the cultural climate of the USA which tends to welcome innovation wholeheartedly. If something has to give, it is more likely to be expenditure budgets than innovation. Moreover, some forms of innovation will reduce rather than raise the overall cost of health care.

In pharmaceuticals, the US market is the world's largest and most receptive to new drugs. Although restrictive cost containment by managed care was feared in the early-1990s when the prophets of doom forecast that it would strangle pharmaceutical innovation, the opposite has occurred. MCOs, in their competitive stance, were able to bargain for substantial discounts from list prices, but found it extremely hard to withhold formulary listing from innovative drugs for fear of tarnishing their reputation for quality care and losing customers.

There are at least 17 different procedures of cost control whereby managed care tries to rein in drug expenditure. It is worth examining these for signs of rationing as distinct from 'normal' cost containment.

Pharmaceutical Cost Control Procedures in US Managed Care

1. prior authorisation
2. prescription by specialists only
3. prescription limited to selected patient groups
4. volume-restricted reimbursement
5. negotiations of conditions for formulary listing
6. delay in formulary decisions
7. higher purchasing discounts
8. higher co-payment or deductibles for patients
9. capitation and risk sharing
10. prescribing guidelines
11. profiling of physicians' prescribing habits
12. 'carve-out' of some or all drugs to external management
13. brand switched to generic at pharmacy
14. pressure on pharmacist to request therapeutic substitution
15. annual or lifetime drug benefit caps for patients

16. staff model control of in-house professionals
17. restricted promotional rep calls on physicians

Five of the 17 procedures are either unequivocal forms of financial control or affect mainly the non-innovative, multiple-source segment of the pharmaceutical market, i.e. procedures 5, 7, 8, 9, and 13.

The remaining 12 procedures are grey-area mechanisms that can be used to target costly forms of innovation.

Prior authorisation (procedure 1) is applied to some expensive new drugs. It means that physicians have to apply for authorisation to prescribe in order to ensure that the patient will receive reimbursement from the insurer. The 'hassle factor' of this procedure deters many doctors from applying for prior authorisation even though refusals are relatively infrequent. In November 1999, a large insurer, United Health Group, announced that it:

> ... will give doctors a final say in medical matters, ending a practice of second-guessing treatment decisions that helped make HMO companies so widely reviled by the public and Congress.

By closing its Utilization Review Division, United Health ended prior authorisation which was not only unpopular with doctors and patients but cost more to administer than it saved on refusals.[29]

Procedures 2 and 3, *Prescription by specialists only* and *Limiting prescribing to selected patient groups* can be defended on medical grounds alone, but can also be used to ration consumption.

Volume-restricted reimbursement (4) which has been widely applied to expensive drugs, is even closer to rationing. It restricts reimbursement to a given number of tablets, prescriptions or refills in a given time period.

Delay in formulary listing decisions (6) arises primarily from attempts to press suppliers for higher discounts. The pharmacy and therapeutics (P&T) committees of MCOs rarely exclude 'medically necessary' new drugs from formularies, but will use delay as an instrument of cost containment.

Prescribing guidelines (10) and *Profiling of physicians' prescribing habits* (11) are designed mainly to ensure good prescribing practice at reasonable cost. Profiling seeks to spot outliers who prescribe excessively or inappropriately. Neither instrument can be classed as rationing unless abused for that purpose.

'Carving out' parts or all of the pharmaceutical sector (12) to external managers is a device to secure tougher or more expert cost control over difficult or expensive treatments. It is sometimes used as a threat: 'we will carve out unless you...', and belongs to the grey area of innovation control. It could be used for rationing purposes.

Pressure on pharmacists to request therapeutic substitution (14) is carrying the fight against high-cost prescribers into the pharmacy. Contract pharmacies will be alerted to expensive prescriptions by pharmacy benefit managers and pressed to ask the prescribing physician whether a lower-cost 'equivalent' (but chemically different) drug could be substituted. Such therapeutic substitution is widespread in hospital settings but illegal in pharmacies without the prescriber's consent. It could be used as a rationing procedure.

Annual or lifetime drug benefit for patients (15) is a form of reimbursement control that does not target innovation specifically but discriminates between patients regardless of need. As such, it can be termed a tool of rationing.

Control of prescribing by physicians who are employees in 'staff-model' MCOs (16) is easier than influencing the contractual behaviour of external group practices of physicians. The intention is to achieve better cost control as well as more appropriate prescribing. It would not normally be regarded as implying rationing.

Finally, *restriction of visits to MCOs by pharmaceutical companies' reps* (17) is designed to reduce the exposure of in-house physicians to drug promotion which has to be channelled through the sieve of a medical or advisory department in the organisation. Whilst a hindrance to promotional market penetration, it cannot be defined as rationing.

Conclusion

Overall, US managed care organisations, acting on behalf of private and public sector insurers, are limited in their ability to ration old or new medical treatments. The limits are set by a blend of regulation, competition, and public opinion. MCOs make energetic efforts to contain costs competitively in order to attract clients, but excessive zeal in that direction has deeply offended public opinion and caused a backlash over alleged neglect of quality. Neither the regulators, nor competitors, nor politicians and the public will allow managed care to convert tough cost containment into healthcare rationing. Grey-area practices, however, are tolerated as long as they do not constitute a blatant downgrading of quality.

The most remarkable trend in US health care is the gradual convergence of public and private sector medicine. Intertwined in the market mechanisms of managed care, this form of symbiosis remains imperfect and defective in some respects, but preserves flexibility and avoids ossification. It also promotes sensitivity to demand in place of top-down planning of supply, and seems to be able to live with the forces of technological innovation even as it struggles to contain their cost.

While access to health care remains a grave problem for a minority of the US population, the patchwork variety of plans for the insured is basically a guarantee that problems will be attacked and solved without having to resort to healthcare rationing.

Part III

T I N A *versus* D O R A

(**T**here **I**s **N**o **A**lternative to rationing health care vs **D**iscover **O**ther **R**ealistic **A**nswers)

With healthcare costs rising steadily in response to demographic pressures, technological advances and popular demand, the view that there is no alternative to rationing has gained ground in several countries, most notably (among those studied here) in the UK, but also in Germany. It is a seductive hypothesis, because it seems to promise fairness and equity, but does it in fact do so? And is it the right solution to the problems of health care in the twenty-first century?

Should Tina have it all her own way, or does Dora deserve at least as much or greater support? In short, are there acceptable and workable alternatives to healthcare rationing?

1

Alternatives to Healthcare Rationing

Les mesures restrictives, difficile à cibler, atteignent souvent en priorité les populations les plus défavorisées.

Restrictive measures are difficult to target and often hit the most deprived first.

Mizrahi, Mizrahi and Sandier[1]

Healthcare rationing should be a last resort when there is truly no alternative. In rich countries, it is a legitimate response to physical scarcity and to little else. Instead, rationing is often regarded as a solution for problems that have been created by excessively tight, man-made budgets.

In a society where nothing else is rationed, the concept of healthcare rationing is a bizarre throwback to the first half of the twentieth century. Then, rationing by top-down planners was often seen as offering a solution to the problems of abject poverty which had been left to fester in the wake of the industrial revolution of the nineteenth century. Allocation and redistribution were potent ideas that could be translated into practical politics, especially under conditions of emergency.

Changes In Society

The planners' dreams collapsed in the rubble of the Berlin Wall at the end of the 1980s. The planned economy in which bureaucrats and expert advisers allocated society's resources to a docile public was revealed as mostly ineffective in countries where the experiment had spanned several generations.

The retention or revival of these principles in the industrialised West, where social conditions are totally different, is indefensible. Yet advocacy of healthcare rationing has continued unabated. Its proponents, like the Bourbons after the French Revolution, have learnt nothing and forgotten nothing. They cannot forget 1945 and they have learnt nothing from 1989.

This is not 1945, and more than a decade has passed since 1989. Folk memories of the dawn of the full-scale welfare state linger on, both in the UK and in France. Germany and France also adhere to the social consensus between employers and unions which has enabled them jointly to exert influence or even direct the course of social security. All the while, the principle of solidarity in health care stands firm as a monument to the founders' dreams.

The ideals on which these West European policies are based have not been invalidated by history, but neither have they been modified or adapted to society's wants and needs at the dawn of the twenty-first century. Moreover, the structures created with the ideals of the years before and after World War II have gradually ossified. Today, they can be viewed as handsome fossils of a bygone era, like steam trains and Hispano-Suizas.

In France, the recent critique of the welfare state in today's social climate (by Denis Kessler[2]), centres on the radical changes that have occurred since the post-war years in *'les risques de l'existence'* ('the risk factors of everyday life'). He cites the example of the wage earners of 1945 whose average life expectation at birth was below their retirement age of 65, whereas today's 'early retirement' pensioners at 55 may well be facing a future life span that is as long as were their years in employment.

The relevance of these thoughts to health care is clear. Ours is an ageing society in which the risk of chronic disease has outpaced the threat of acute infections that loomed so large in 1945; where technology and the demand for it are advancing arm in arm; and where the borderline between preventive lifestyles and the treatment of illness is becoming blurred.

Compared with 1945, today's industrialised or post-industrial society is also one in which health care is nationally affordable if people want it enough and are willing to pay for it by a variety of methods. It is a society in which individual responsibility should begin to play a more prominent role than in the social climate of 1945 when protection against the risk factors of everyday life was rightly seen as the key priority. To avoid the issue of greater personal responsibility today by resorting to rationing in rich countries is inadmissible.

Solidarity In Need Of An Update

The principle of solidarity in health care stipulates that society will provide for the care of those who are unable to provide for themselves. Together with the principle of universal coverage, solidarity forms the foundation on which European health care has been built.

Both principles remain valid. To abandon either and move towards an American-style system without universal coverage (although with a greater emphasis on solidarity in the USA now than there was in the past) would be politically suicidal in the European Union.

There is, however, room for updating both principles, or at least dusting them down and removing the cobwebs of misinterpretation that have gradually obscured their original meanings. *Universal coverage* means that the entire population is entitled to and receives health care. It does not mean that everybody is entitled to receive everything in the way of health care free at the point of use. Similarly, *solidarity* means looking after those who cannot look after themselves. It does not imply an obligation to supply healthcare freebies to everyone else, including those who are quite capable of paying or contributing towards the cost of health services.

The claim that everything must be free for everybody all the time has perverted the purpose of solidarity and universal coverage. That is disputed by many who insist that, having paid their taxes or social insurance contributions, they *are* now entitled to everything free all the time. That notion, too, dates back to 1945 when health care had only just emerged from its nineteenth century chrysalis. The 'wonder drug' era had begun with sulphonamides and penicillin but was not yet in full swing. Surgery was still relatively primitive, doctors were gods and patients knew their place. In short, it was a time when universal coverage was 'manna from heaven'.

One is grateful to heaven for manna. One does not demand that heaven despatch it gift-wrapped by express courier. If one did, a suitable contribution towards postage and packing would be regarded as appropriate and would not cause political uproar—except in European health care.

The claim that payment of tax or social insurance absolves the payer from all financial obligations at the point of use is irrational. *The purpose of these contributions is not to absolve the contributor but to cover those who are unable to contribute.* That principle remains valid. To extend it to 'everything free for everybody all the time' is evidently unsustainable without rationing, so that the health care that is then made available is levelled down to what is affordable 'free'.

Future advances in surgery and in medical and pharmaceutical technology alone will make such a set of assumptions irrelevant and drive changes in the rules of solidarity and universal coverage. Past advances, however spectacular, are minimal compared with those that are to come in the first half of the twenty-first century. They will not be cheap and although some forms of innovation will reduce the cost of overall health care (e.g. drugs that replace surgery and hospitalisation), it would be unrealistic to believe that healthcare expenditure will fall under the impact of innovation. If the cost of new technology is to be financially sustainable, will European society tolerate major increases in taxation? And if not, must it be rationing or are there alternatives?

A Hierarchy Of Alternatives To Healthcare Rationing

The alternatives can be considered under four headings:

1. Redefinition of the solidarity principle
2. Diversification of funding
3. Diversification of choice
4. Greater individual responsibility for health

1. Redefinition of the solidarity principle

As discussed above, this is a prerequisite for attitudinal change. It will not of itself produce major savings, although higher user charges for those who can afford them would help to ease the budgetary problems from which rationing springs.

The main objective in redefining solidarity is to remind taxpayers and contributors to social insurance that they are not paying for a lifetime of 'free' health care, but in order to provide adequate care for those who are unable to contribute. Without such a change in outlook, TINA will win the day. At that point, There Is No Alternative to rationing—as the UK has already discovered and Germany is afraid of discovering.

2. Diversification of funding

Designing the rules under which people can buy health care outside of a budget-controlled system, either through private insurance or with cash, is a deep and subtle issue of economics, ethics, and politics. The right answer almost certainly varies from country to country and from time to time, but the right limit on such 'outside-the-system' purchases is never 'none'.[3]

Diversification of funding is a necessary corollary of the redefinition of solidarity. Instead of relying solely or almost exclusively on the state, additional sources need to be tapped. These can take the form of supplementary insurance (filling gaps in public sector reimbursement) or that of comprehensive private health insurance for those who wish to opt out of public sector coverage. That does not mean dismantling public health services. On the contrary, it will help to relieve their financial plight, whilst regulation can ensure that the public system remains stable and the supplementary sources remain supplementary. That private health insurance alone cannot replace public coverage in modern society is demonstrated by the increasing convergence and cooperation between the two in the USA (see Part II-7).

France has shown how its *assurance complémentaire* can help to achieve and maintain high levels of healthcare consumption with high standards of quality and outcomes, in response to popular demand. There, supplementary insurance works side by side with a public sector system that also performs well but is in a permanent state of financial crisis. France likes DORA and has no time for TINA.

The 1940s dogma of maintaining the purity of public funding through thick and thin can only lead in TINA's direction: no alternative to rationing. That is the price of egalitarian idealism: equity is enforced by levelling down. Solidarity does not require absolute equity in health care any more than total equity in food, clothing and other necessities of life. It requires adequate provision for those who are unable to provide it for themselves. Modern society in an ageing post-industrial world demands more than that as a consumer option in health care. If that demand, too, is to be satisfied, healthcare funding needs to be diversified.

3. Diversification of choice

TINA, goddess of rationing, is the commander of allocation and the enemy of choice: choice of insurer, choice of plan, choice of physician, choice of specialist, choice of hospital venue, choice of treatment. TINA will have none of these.

Choice, which patients will be demanding more and more insistently as the twenty-first century unfolds, can drive market forces (as in the USA), or it can be accommodated within highly controlled systems (as in France). In between free markets and tight controls, choice can be offered by mixed health insurance systems as in Switzerland, where every patient must be given a federally determined basic range of benefits but can choose additional benefits at various levels of risk and cost-sharing.

For those who wish to condemn this as 'two-tier medicine', it is suggested that they take a trip to Switzerland first. The level of obligatory coverage of basic medical care in Switzerland is set high. In August 2000, the President of the Federal Commission for Basic Issues in Health Insurance (*Eidgenössische Kommission für Grundsatzfragen der Krankenversicherung*) declared that 'there is no necessity to ration medical provision in Switzerland ... That applies also to expensive treatments for which no cheaper equivalent alternatives are available. The new Federal constitution clearly prohibits discrimination in medical provision in accordance with the Health Insurance Law. Necessary medical treatment must be accessible to all.' Limitation of choice, for example by way of waiting lists, should be imposed only in emergencies or for reasons of temporary shortages in resources, and in organ transplantation where demand exceeds supply.[4]

Swiss experience demonstrates that the solidarity principle is quite capable of operating with choice after the provision of 'necessary' care has been satisfied. While diversified choice is an intrinsic component of market-based systems, it can also help to develop the diversification of funding, because it provides patients with the incentive of increased benefits for higher payments, insured or at the point of use.

4. Greater individual responsibility for health

This may well prove to be the most difficult healthcare challenge of the twenty-first century. Preventive lifestyles are socially desirable and would help to avoid unnecessary medical interventions. Prevention is, however, difficult to achieve and requires education rather than exhortation. Can it be linked, by incentives or penalties, to society's judgment of whether or not patients are to blame for their condition?

Greater individual responsibility for health itself and for the cost of care are potentially important alternatives to rationing. They also present unattractive ethical choices. Should society have to pay for those who are wilfully ruining their health? On the other hand, are we going to have a Health Police with informers, tribunals and court cases to identify and distinguish the unregenerate smoker from those who are victims of lung cancer for 'permissible' reasons and may qualify for free treatment?

It looks as though the incentive route and the educational mode will be more practical and more acceptable approaches than the pillory for health 'criminals'.

The responsible and responsive patient has much to contribute to the development of affordable health care within a redefined framework of solidarity, based on a variety of sources of funds and offering choice. Such systems, in which the public and private sectors intertwine, can live with the application of 'normal' methods of cost containment. They are not obliged to ration health care.

2

Options for the Way Ahead in the United Kingdom

When it comes to health care, no government or public is likely to opt for revolution ... The issues in health care are too complex and unpredictable for even the most foolhardy anarchist to tackle.
                                                                            Robert G. Geursen[1]

The National Health Service—like that other venerable institution, the London underground—is badly in need of a refit, but the last thing that the public wants is for anarchists to blow it up. *Tabula rasa*, the sick fancy of extremists, is not a practical proposition. Britain cannot and will not start again from scratch.

Although the NHS is perpetually underfunded, the cure for that ailment is primarily a political task. Finance is a key component of the *problem*, not of the answer. Money could be raised in any number of ways if the political will to do so were firm enough and sufficiently confident of electoral support.

Neither of these pre-conditions seems to exist in the UK. The political debate, like an ancient gramophone record, has been stuck for decades in a groove of outdated dogma. It is politically correct in the UK to assert that:

i)   all (or nearly all) health care must be channelled *via* the NHS

ii) all (or nearly all) of it must be free at the point of use

iii) the answer to the problems arising from underfunding is health-care rationing

Whereas the public believes in the first two tenets of the faith, the majority of healthcare experts appear to believe in all three. It is therefore pertinent to examine, first of all, the validity of 'dogmatic solutions', i.e. those that can be accommodated within the confines of received opinion.

'In-dogma' Solutions

To satisfy the first two requirements (a monopoly, free at the point of use) will, in the long run, require a combination of higher personal taxation, sustained and rapid growth of the economy, the withdrawal of funds from other sectors of public expenditure for re-allocation to the NHS, and a radical upgrade of the efficiency of the health service.

Higher taxation

Higher personal taxation has meant death at the ballot box for the past 20 years. With the public continuing to demand 'more money for the NHS', it is conceivable that a form of hypothecated taxation, directly allocated to the NHS, might now win public acquiescence up to a point. The Treasury dislikes the precedent set by hypothecation, but that is one of the few public battles that can still be fought behind closed doors.

> Cigarette taxes will rise by five per cent above inflation from tonight ... with every penny of the extra revenue going—as promised—to funding our hospitals and the National Health Service.
>
> (Chancellor's Budget 2000 speech, 21 March 2000)

It is a small step in the direction of hypothecation. The main drive to improve funding of the NHS in 'Budget 2000' is a commitment to increase health spending over the next five years by 35 per cent in *real* terms. This is to be financed from current and projected budget surpluses. As long as these persist, higher personal taxation imposed specifically to provide more health care can probably be avoided. The question remains: how long can these conditions last?

Sustained and rapid economic growth

With increasing globalisation, the national economy is no longer dependent on national management alone. Events in the world at large can upset the best-laid plans almost overnight. The theme of *'sustained and rapid economic growth'* is the melodic lure of future music. It may seem to solve problems for a while. For health care to rely on an indefinite 'Goldilocks scenario' in an increasingly silver-haired society smacks of fairyland and happy ends in comic opera. As Gilbert and Sullivan put it in *The Mikado*:

> *The flowers that bloom in the spring,*
> *Tra-la,*
> *Breathe promise of merry sunshine.*
> *As we merrily dance and we sing,*
> *Tra-la,*
> *We welcome the hope that they bring,*
> *Tra-la,*
> *Of a summer of roses and wine.*

Tra-la, indeed.

Re-allocation of public funds to the NHS

It is difficult to assess the realistic prospects of intra-budgetary transfers without the documentation that is at the Chancellor's disposal. However, to judge by the desperate cries for more public money to be poured into education, public transport, the armed forces, and Uncle Tom Cobley and All, the prospects of 'robbing Peter to pay Paul' are dubious alternatives to budget surpluses.

Upgrading the efficiency of the NHS
(see 'The efficiency delusion', Part II-4)

In a health care world of extreme uncertainty, one thing seems certain: higher efficiency, whilst desirable and always feasible, can neither solve the underlying crisis of the NHS nor make a prime contribution to its resolution. In some respects, the efficiency drive in the NHS has already undermined the quality of the service, as it has done in US managed care.

The NHS Plan (July 2000)

Following the government's commitment to increased funding in 'Budget 2000', *The NHS Plan: a Plan for Investment, a Plan for Reform* was presented to Parliament in July 2000.[2] At long last, it acknowledges the need to address the chronic underfunding of the service. The Plan also restates the Government's 'vision' of the NHS and proposes to reform its procedures and upgrade its performance in accordance with national standards and targets set by the Department of Health.

In relation to healthcare *rationing* (the subject most relevant to this study), the projected massive injection of funds is to be welcomed, and it has been welcomed by most healthcare partners and commentators. No other way of *rapidly* channelling badly needed additional funds of this magnitude into UK health care is realistically conceivable.

The plan is weakest where it aims to be strongest: in its 'vision' and performance targets. Government vision of health care remains firmly lodged on the ideological horizon of 1945. The Plan pays little more than lip service to the realities of twenty-first century medical, scientific and social change. On performance targets, the Plan condemns 'over-centralisation' but promptly proceeds to set centralised targets reminiscent of mid-twentieth century top-down planning.

Can the NHS Plan end the rationing climate of health care in the United Kingdom?

In the short term, it can probably alleviate its most acute manifestations. In the medium term, the resource targets may be both insufficient and difficult to achieve on the planned time scale.

For example, there is a target for 9,500 additional practising physicians (consultants and GPs) in the UK by 2004.

Fact: in 1997, there were 75,800 more practising physicians in France than in the UK, for the same population size.

Even allowing for a substantial surplus over necessary resources in France, the planned increase in the UK seems inadequate for an unrationed modern health service. It is symptomatic of the Plan's reluctance to face facts that conflict with its vision.

The Executive Summary states that the Plan

> has examined other forms of healthcare and found them wanting. The systems used by other countries do not provide a route to better healthcare.

This remarkable assertion misses the point. All *systems* are imperfect. Neither social insurance, nor tax funding, nor private health insurance, nor supplementary coverage alone will provide the solution to the problems of healthcare funding and performance. In effect, there is no such thing as The Solution.

One size no longer fits all, if indeed it ever did. The complexity of modern society demands a multiplicity of partial solutions for different circumstances, flexible enough to change as circumstances alter.

To assert that *'the systems used by other countries do not provide a route to better healthcare'* ignores evidence that other countries of comparable economic status have allocated a more intensive input of resources to health care and—irrespective of their systems—appear to be producing significantly better health outcomes in many areas of care.

Overall, the 'In-Dogma' scenario, including the NHS Plan, can buy time but does not look promising as a means of overcoming the fundamental long-term problems of the NHS. Rationing, which the Plan rejects conceptually in terms of reducing public sector health care to a 'core service', can be expected to continue *de facto* in the NHS under its new Plan.

'Beyond-Dogma' Solutions

The need for structural alternatives 'beyond the dogma' is underlined by the fact that healthcare expenditure in the UK is *abnormally* low by comparison with neighbouring nations, and *abnormally* dependent on public funds (see Part II-1). This makes it hard to fulfil the demands even of the relatively undemanding British public.

If rationing is to be eliminated (other than under conditions of unavoidable shortage as in organ transplantation), some taboos will have to be broken. It is essentially a question of whether the sanctity of the dogma will continue to be allowed to prevail over self-evident practical needs.

The question is not whether the NHS is to be replaced but whether healthcare resources can be further increased and diversified. The demand for health care is rising ineluctably with an ageing population, more assertive patients, and major impending advances in medical science and technology. None of these factors respond to the ups-and-downs of the economic cycle. To cope with the problems of a less buoyant economy, it must be prudent to supplement NHS healthcare funding with additional, independent sources that will be less critically dependent on the performance of the economy or the level of government borrowing.

Other countries have produced partial solutions by retreating from idealistic perfectionism. France has used supplementary insurance as a buffer between an overburdened national insurance scheme and public demand for both quality and quantity in health care. Germany has permitted the higher income groups to opt out of Statutory Health Insurance and obtain private coverage instead. The USA, whilst not solving the inequality of access to health care, has allowed substantial convergence between the public and the private sector so that the efficiency of managed care could be harnessed for cost containment in Medicare and Medicaid. Switzerland has chosen mandatory basic insurance by the public sector with a variety of public and private choices for additional coverage.

None of these systems is perfect. French health care operates in a maze of control agreements between government and the healthcare partners and rejects market forces altogether. Germany has hedged the competitive climate which its reforms appear to encourage by so many obstacles that the system is in danger of sliding into a rationing mode which neither government nor insurers nor providers nor the public want. The USA has failed to provide universal coverage and is in the throes of a political battle between the agents of efficiency (managed care) and the guardians of patients' rights. Switzerland, whose system is probably the clearest signpost to a compromise between solidarity, public sector control, and market forces, complains that its system remains unduly wasteful and inefficient, although it provides excellent health care.

None of these countries have chosen *rationing* as the answer to their problems. In most respects, their systems have retained a greater level of public satisfaction and have met the major healthcare challenges of our day with a more consistent performance and better outcomes than the UK.

'Pluralism' —A Clutch Of Solutions

> We must distinguish between the moral idealism of the NHS aspiration and its practical results, and be prepared to make changes where they are necessary. Through greater pluralism, we can indeed improve the access to high-quality health care as a whole.[3]

There is no single solution to the problems of the National Health Service. There is no panacea that will work a miracle overnight. In the politics of health care, there are no public funds that will provide the NHS with adequate budgets to furnish a high-grade modern service as a public monopoly in the long run.

The public has a right to demand choice and will be driven to do so by impending changes in the risks of everyday life. In an ageing society, with more and more single person households, health will acquire an even higher priority for individuals than it has already. For those of working age, health is the passport to employment; for the elderly, it is the prerequisite for an independent lifestyle. Neither the employed nor the retired can fall back on the extended, or even the nuclear, family as in the past. Rationed health care will not, in reality, share the burdens of sickness and disability, but will increase them.

Why should the public put up with inadequate health care for the sake of upholding the ideological dogma of their great-grandfathers?

Pluralism means horses for courses. There is room for a performing NHS and there is room for supplementary forms of health insurance. There is room for obligatory provision and there is room for extras. There is room for choice, for incentives, for risk sharing, for competition, and perhaps for penalties. There is room for user charges and for exemption from user charges. There is room for regarding health care as a basic right, and there is room for taking greater personal and financial responsibility for one's own health.

There is also room for adopting some aspects of the pluralistic experience of comparable countries and adapting them to the cultural needs and preferences of the United Kingdom.

The only aspects for which there should be no room in modern society are the denial of health care to the needy, and rationing.

A plurality of systems with a plurality of choice is inescapable unless the answer to the question *'Why ration health care?'* is to be *'Why not!'*

Why not?

Because rationed health care will not be able to cope with the risks of everyday life in the twenty-first century.

Notes

Part I
1: The R-word in Healthcare Politics

1 Kneeshaw, J., 'What does the public think about rationing? A review of the evidence', in New, B. (ed.), *Rationing: Talk and Action in Health Care*, Kings Fund, London: BMJ Publishing Group, 1997.

2 Klein, R., 'Puzzling out priorities: why we must acknowledge that rationing is a political process', *British Medical Journal,* 317, 959, 10 October 1998.

3 Ham, C., 'Synthesis: what can we learn from international experience?', in Maxwell, R.J. (ed.), *Rationing Health Care*, Churchill Livingstone, *Brit. Medical Bull*, 51(4), 1995, 819-30.

2: Crossing the Border

1 Geursen, R., 'Script: a pharmaceutical executive looks at the question of equity', in *EIU Healthcare International*, 2nd quarter 1999, The Economist Intelligence Unit, 1999.

2 Spiers, J., *The Realities of Rationing: 'Priority Setting' in the NHS*, London: IEA Health & Welfare Unit, 1999.

3 New, B. and Le Grand, J., *Rationing in the NHS: Principles and Pragmatism*, London: King's Fund, 1996.

4 Spiers, *The Realities of Rationing*, 1999.

5 Cooper, M. H., 'Core services and the New Zealand health reforms', in Maxwell, R.J. (ed.), *Rationing Health Care*, Churchill Livingston, *Brit. Medical Bull*. 51(4), 1995.

6 Green, D. and Casper, L., *Denial, Delay & Dilution: The Impact of NHS Rationing on Heart Disease and Cancer*, London: IEA Health & Welfare Unit, 2000.

7 Klein, R., 'Defining a package of NHS healthcare services: the case against', in New, B. (ed.), *Rationing: Talk and Action in Health Care*, King's Fund, London: BMJ Publishing Group 1997.

8 Cueni, T., *Rationalisieren oder Rationieren?*, Basel: Interpharma, 1997.

9 Bosanquet, N., *A Successful National Health Service*, London: Adam Smith Institute, 1999.

3: Symptoms and Tools

1 Conan Doyle, A., 'The Adventure of Silver Blaze', *Strand Magazine*, December 1892.

2 Audit Commission, *A Prescription for Improvement*, London: HMSO, 1994.

3   French *numerus clausus* restrictions for medical students are now to be reversed in order to avoid a *future* shortage of doctors.

4   Donelan, K., Blendon, R.J., Schoen, C., Davis, K. and Binns, K., 'The cost of health system change: public discontent in five nations', *Health Affairs* 14(3), 206-216, May/June 1998.

4: When Rationing is Inevitable

1   The *Times*, 28 January 2000.

2   Harper, A.M. *et al*, Clin. Transplant. 1998 , 73-90.

3   Helderman, J. H. and Goral, S., 'The allocation of cadaveric kidneys', *New England Journal of Medicine*, 341 (19) 1468-9, 4 November 1999.

4   *Health Care Financing Review*, 1998 Statistical Supplement.

5   Carey, J., 'DHHS sets out modified rules for giving sickest patients priority for organ transplants', *CQ Weekly*, 23 October 1999, 2530.

6   Zenios, S.A. *et al*, 'Evidence-based organ allocation', *American Journal of Medicine*, 107, 52-61, July 1999.

7   Neuberger, J. *et al*, 'Assessing priorities for the allocation of donor liver grafts: survey of public and clinicians', *BMJ* 317, 172-5, 18 July 1998.

8   Neuberger, 'Assessing priorities for the allocation of donor liver grafts', 1998.

Part II
1: Health Expenditure and Resources

1   Leidl, R., 'Europäische Integration und Entwicklung der Gesundheitsausgaben', in ZEW Wirtschaftsanalysen 33, *Entwicklung und Perspektiven der Sozialversicherung*, Baden-Baden: Nomos-Verlag, 1999.

2   Schieber, G.J., Poullier, J-P. and Greenwald, C.M., 'Health system performance in the OECD countries 1980-1992', *Health Affairs* 13, 100-112, Fall 1994.

3   Anderson, G.F. and Poullier, J-P., 'Health spending, access and outcomes: trends in the industrialized countries', *Health Affairs*, 18(3), 178-192, May-June 1999.

2: Morbidity and Outcomes

1   Anderson, G.F. and Poullier, J-P., 'Health spending, access and outcomes: trends in the industrialized countries', *Health Affairs*, 18(3), 178-192, May-June 1999.

2   Green, D.G. and Casper, L., *Delay, Denial and Dilution: The Impact of NHS Rationing on Heart Disease and Cancer*, London: IEA Health & Welfare Unit, 2000.

3: Satisfaction and Opinion Surveys

1   Royal Commission on Long-Term Care, *With Respect to Old Age: Long Term Care—Rights and Responsibilities*, Research Volume I, Cm 4192-II/1, London, March 1999.

2   Mossialos, E., 'Citizens' views of health systems in the 15 member states of the European Union', *Health Economics*, 6, 109-116, 1997.

3   Quoted in Royal Commission, *With Respect to Old Age*, 1999.

4   OECD, *Health Data 99*, various sources quoted in 'Satisfaction with healthcare systems'.

5   Blendon, R. *et al*, 'Who has the best healthcare system? A second look', *Health Affairs*, 14(4), 220-230, 1995.

6   Donelan, K., Blendon, R.J. *et al*, 'The cost of health system change: public discontent in five nations', *Health Affairs* 18(3), 206-216, May/June 1999.

7   Mossialos, E., 'Citizens' views of health systems in the 15 member states of the European Union', *Health Economics*, 6, 109-116, 1997.

8   Donelan, Blendon *et al*, 'The cost of health system change', 1999.

9   Donelan, Blendon *et al*, 'The cost of health system change', 1999.

10 Donelan, Blendon *et al*, 'The cost of health system change', 1999.

11 Payer, L., *Medicine and Culture*, New York: Henry Holt & Co., 1988.

12 CREDES (Centre de Recherche, d'Etude et de Documentation en Economie de la Santé), 'Questions d'économie de la santé', *Bulletin d'information en économie de la santé*, No. 24, December 1999.

13 Haut Comité de la Santé Publique, 'La Santé en France 1994-1998', Ministère de l'Emploi et de la Solidarité, La Documentation Française, Paris, September 1998.

14 Royal Commission, *With Respect to Old Age,* 1999.

15 Royal Commission, *With Respect to Old Age,*1999.

4: The United Kingdom: A Rationing Climate

1   Mossialos, E. and Le Grand, J., *Health Care and Cost Containment in the European Union*, Ashgate Publishing Ltd, 1999.

2   Ham, C., 'Resources and rationing in the NHS', in Macpherson, G. (ed.), *Our NHS: A Celebration of 50 Years*, London: BMJ Books, 1998.

3   Mossialos and Le Grand, *Health Care and Cost Containment in the European Union*, 1999.

4   Mossialos and Le Grand, *Health Care and Cost Containment in the European Union*, 1999.

5   Donelan, K., Blendon, R.J. *et al*, 'The cost of health system change: public discontent in five nations', *Health Affairs* 18(3), 206-216, May/June 1999.

6   Handelsblatt, 'Fischer verspricht stabile Beiträge', 1 July 1999.

7   Bosanquet, N., 'Exposing symptoms of innovation phobia and the effectiveness gap', *British Journal of Health Care Management*, 11(11), November 1998.

8   Donelan, Blendon *et al*, 'The cost of health system change', 1999.

9   Donelan, Blendon *et al*, 'The cost of health system change', 1999.

10 Laing & Buisson, *Laing's Healthcare Market Review 1999-2000*, 12th edition, London, 1999.

11 Central Office of Information, Department of Health, 'NHS Performance: The New NHS Performance Tables 1997/98'.

12 Headline, *Sunday Times*, 11 July 1999.

13 *Sunday Times*, 16 January 2000.

14 Letter to the Editor, The *Times*, 20 January 2000, from a senior clergyman, St. Paul's Cathedral.

15 The *Times*, 10 January 2000.

16 *Financial Times*, 22 March 2000.

17 Letter to the Editor, The *Times*, from Professors Sir John Vane, G.V.R. Born and L. L. Iverson, 15 January 1999.

18 Beard, K., Forrester, E. *et al*, 'Systems and strategies for managing the drugs budget in Glasgow', *BMJ*, 317, 1378-1381, 14 November 1998.

19 Brown, P.J., 'NICE: seriously nasty but welcome nevertheless', *Scrip*, November 1999, pp. 3-4.

20 Secretary of State for Health, White Paper, *The New NHS: Modern, Dependable*, Cm. 3807, London: Stationery Office, December 1997.

21 *Scrip*, 'NICE clears taxanes for breast cancer', 21 June 2000, p. 2.

22 *Scrip*, 'Seven appeals to NICE on beta-interferon', 30 August 2000, p. 3.

23 The *Times*, 22 June 2000.

24 *Daily Telegraph*, 9 February 1999.

25 Pharma Pricing and Reimbursement, Conference Report, 'Benign neglect by UK doctors inhibits use of newer drugs', May 1999, pp. 104-08.

5: France: Crisis in Plenty

1 Kessler, D., 'L'avenir de la protection sociale', *Commentaires* No. 87, Autumn 1999.

2 Polton, D., 'La maîtrise des dépenses de santé', *Le Concours Médical*, 121(23), 1874-1887, 12 June 1999.

3 Duriez, M., Lancry, P.J. *et al*, 'Le système de santé en France', *Que Sais-je?*, No. 3066, Presses Universitaires de France, 1996.

4 Delorme, J., 'Le Rapport Mougeot, I – Le bilan du système de santé en France', *Le Concours Médical*, 121(7), 20 February 1999.

5 Chabrun-Robert, C. 'La démographie médicale et le revenu des médecins libéraux en 1997', *Le Concours Médical*, 121(9), 659-663, 6 March 1999.

6 Chabrun-Robert, 'La démographie médicale et le revenu des médecins libéraux en 1997', 1999.

7 Cognat, C. 'Edouard-Herriot en mal d'anaesthésistes', *Le Progrès*, 19 October 1999.

8 Economist Intelligence Unit, 'EIU global outlook—France', 1999.

9 Lancry, P-J. and Sandier, S., 'Vingt années de remèdes pour le système de santé en France', *CREDES*, September 1996.

10 Taupin, B., 'Sécurité Sociale: un excédent modeste pour 2000', *Le Figaro Economie*, 22 September 1999.

11 Bader, J-P., 'L'ONDAM face à la mutation de la santé', *Le Quotidien du Médecin*, 25 November 1999, pp. 21-22.

12 Bader, 'L'ONDAM face à la mutation de la santé', 1999.

13 Gabillat, C., 'Dossier Accord Sectoriel: Noël Renaudin – une volonté de transparence et de concertation', *Pharmaceutiques* No. 69, September 1999, pp. 52-55.

14 Le Pen, C., 'Le Cours Nouveau de la Politique du Médicament', reprinted in *Tableau de Bord*, Carré Castan Consultants, 10 December 1999.

15 Bonneau, A., 'Réevaluation I—La phase contradictoire', Pharmaceutiques No. 69, September 1999, pp. 10-11.

16 'Liste des molécules entrant dans la composition des produits d'AMM centralisée non commercialisées en France', *Pharmaceutiques*, 75, March 2000, p. 15.

17 Lancry and Sandier, 'Vingt années de remèdes pour le système de santé en France', 1996.

18 Graham, R., 'An end to patronage', *Financial Times*, 20 January 2000.

19 Lancry and Sandier, 'Vingt années de remèdes pour le système de santé en France', 1996.

20 Bocognano, A., Dumesnil, S. *et al*, 'Santé, soins et protection sociale en 1998', Biblio No. 1282, *CREDES*, Paris, December 1999.

21 Ministère de l'Emploi et de la Solidarité, 'Comptes nationaux de la santé', Rapport juillet 1997.

22 Duriez, Lancry *et al*, 'Le système de santé en France', 1996.

6: Germany: *Achtung!* Rationing Alert!

1   Cassel, D., 'Eine amputierte zustimmungsfreie Gesundheitsreform ist keine Lösung', *Handelsblatt*, 6 December 1999, p. 2.

2   Ärzte-Zeitung, 'Europäische Gesundheitssysteme und Pharma-Märkte', Ärzte-Zeitung Verlagsges. mbH, Neu Isenburg, December 1998.

3   Lankers, C.H.R., 'Erfolgsfaktoren von Managed Care auf europäischen Märkten', WIdO 37, Wissenschaftliches Institut der AOK, Bonn, 1997.

4   Advisory Council for Concerted Action in Health Care, 'The healthcare system in Germany—cost factor and branch of the future', Volume I, Special Report, Summary, Bonn 1996.

5   Graig, L.A., *Health of Nations*, 3rd edition, Congressional Quarterly Inc., Washington DC, 1999.

6   Ärzte-Zeitung, 'Europäische Gesundheitssysteme und Pharma-Märkte', Ärzte-Zeitung Verlagsges. mbH, Neu Isenburg, December 1998.

7   Hanson, F., 'Teure patienten unerwünscht', *Die Zeit*, 11 November 1999.

8   Schwabe, U., 'Überblick über die Arzneiverordnungen im Jahre 1998', in Schwabe, U. and Paffrath, D. (eds.), *Arzneiverordnungs-Report 1999*, Springer, Berlin 2000; Also, Schröder, H. and Selke, G. W., 'Der Arzneimittelmarkt in der Bundesrepublik Deutschland', in *Arzneiverordnungs-Report 1999*.

9   Rahner, E. 'Lebhafter Streit um das KBV-Notprogramm gegen Überschreitungen der Arzneibudgets', *Die Pharmazeutische Industrie* 61(8), 159-161, August 1999.

10 Ehlers, A.P.F., 'Das Fünf-Punkte-Notprogramm der Kassenärztliche Bundesvereinigung. Das Ende der Dialogbereitschaft?', *Die Pharmazeutische Industrie* 61(8), 714-715, August 1999.

11 Rahner, 'Lebhafter Streit um das KBV-Notprogramm gegen Überschreitungen der Arzneibudgets', 1999.

12 Kassenärztliche Bundesvereinigung, 'Gemeinsames Aktionsprogramm zur Einhaltung der Arznei-und Heilmittelbudgets 1999', August 1999.

13 *Handelsblatt*, 'Fischer verspricht stabile Beiträge', 1 July 1999, p. 4.

14 *Handelsblatt*, 'Fischers Notgesetz im Vermittlungsausschuss', 3 December 1999, p. 3.

15 Zok, K., 'Anforderungen an die Gesetzliche Krankenversicherung —Einschätzungen und Erwartungen aus Sicht der Versicherten', WIdO 43, Wissenschaftliches Institut der AOK, Bonn, December 1999.

16 Zok, 'Anforderungen an die Gesetzliche Krankenversicherung —Einschätzungen und Erwartungen aus Sicht der Versicherten', 1999.

7: The USA: The Power to Make Choices

1 Pauly, M.V., 'Competition in the market for health services and insurance, with special reference to the United States', in Giersch, H. (ed.), *Merits and Limits of Markets*, Berlin: Springer, 1998.

2 Poisal, J.A., Murray, L.A. *et al*, 'Prescription drug coverage and spending for Medicare beneficiaries', *Health Care Financing Review* 20(3), 15-27,Spring 1999.

3 Iglehart, J.K., 'The American healthcare system—Medicaid', *New England Journal of Medicine*, 340(5), 403-408, 4 February 1999.

4 Levit, K., Cowan, C., Lazenby, H. *et al*, 'Health spending in 1998: signals of change', *Health Affairs* 19(1), 124-132, January/February 2000.

5 Levit, Cowan, Lazenby *et al*, 'Health spending in 1998', 2000.

6 Braden, B.R., Cowan, C.,Lazenby, H.C. *et al*, 'National Health expenditures 1997', *Health Care Financing Review* 20(1), 83-126, Fall 1998.

7 Graig, L.A., *Health of Nations*, 3rd edition, Congressional Quarterly Inc, Washington DC, 1999.

8 Iglehart, 'The American healthcare system—Medicaid', 1999.

9 Ya-chen, T.S., 'Effect of insurance on prescription drug use by ESRD beneficiaries', *Health Care Financing Review* 20(3), 39-53, Spring 1999.

10 Moon, M., *Medicare Now and in the Future*, 2nd edition, Urban Institute Press, Washington DC, 1997.

11 Moon, *Medicare Now and in the Future*, 1997.

12 Moon, M., *Medicare Now and in the Future*, 1997.

13 National Pharmaceutical Council, 'Pharmaceutical Benefits under State Medical Assistance Programs', Reston, Va, November 1997.

14 National Pharmaceutical Council, 'Pharmaceutical Benefits under State Medical Assistance Programs', 1997.

15 Maggio, C.O., Testimony before the House Sub-Committee on Human Resources and Intergovernmental Relations, on 'State Medicaid Formularies: Cost saving measure or second-class medicine?', 103rd Congress, 9 June 1993, Washington DC: US Government Printing Office, 1995.

16 Bodenheimer, T., 'The Oregon health plan—lessons for the nation', Part I, *New England Journal of Medicine* 337(9), 651-655, 28 August 1997.

17 Bodenheimer, 'The Oregon health plan—lessons for the nation', 1997.

18 Klein, R., 'Defining a package of healthcare services the NHS is responsible for—the case against', in New, B. (ed.), *Rationing—Talk and Action in Health Care*, BMJ Publishing Group, 1997.

19 Bodenheimer, 'The Oregon health plan—lessons for the nation', 1997.

20 Iglehart, 'The American healthcare system—Medicaid', 1999.

21 Levit, Cowan, Lazenby *et al*, 'Health spending in 1998', 2000.

22 Braden, Cowan, Lazenby *et al*, 'National health expenditures 1997', 1998.

23 Poisal, Murray *et al*, 'Prescription drug coverage and spending for Medicare beneficiaries', 1999.

24 Taylor, A., Carey, M.A. *et al*, 'What the Budget Bill does', *CQ Weekly Report*, 13 December 1997, pp. 3082-84.

25 Redwood, H., *Pharmapolitics 2000*, Felixstowe, England: Oldwicks Press Limited, 1997.

26 'The lowdown on HMOs', *Business and Health*, October 1998, p. 12.

27 Pauly, 'Competition in the market for health services and insurance, with special reference to the United States', 1998.

28 Pauly, 'Competition in the market for health services and insurance, with special reference to the United States', 1998.

29 Burton, T.M., 'United Health to end ruling on treatments', *Wall St Journal*, 9 November 1999, p. A3.

Part III
1: Alternatives to Healthcare Rationing

1 Mizrahi, An., Mizrahi, Ar. and Sandier, S. 'Quel système de santé demain?', *Le Concours Médical*, 121(24), 1965-8, 19 June 1999.

2   Kessler, D., *L'Avenir de la Protection Sociale*, *Commentaires* No. 87, 619-632, autumn 1999.

3   Aaron, H., 'Thinking about healthcare finance: some propositions' in 'Healthcare reform—the will to change', *Health Policy Studies*, No. 8, OECD Paris 1996.

4   Piller, O., reported by Schweizerische Depeschenagentur, 'Umgang mit teuren medizinischen Leistungen: Grundsatzkommission gegen Rationierung—Rationalisierung ja', 24 August 2000. (Author's translation of news report.)

2: Options for the Way Ahead in the United Kingdom

1   Geursen, R.G., 'Script—a pharmaceutical executive looks at the question of equity', EIU Healthcare International, 2nd Quarter 1999, The Economist Intelligence Unit, 1999.

2   Secretary of State for Health, *The NHS Plan: a Plan for Investment, a Plan for Reform*, Cm 4818-I, London: Stationery Office, July 2000.

3   Bosanquet, N., *A Successful National Health Service*, London: Adam Smith Institute, 1999.

Index